With careful thought and gentle intention, Aundi is a trusted guide who distills what she's learned as a trauma-informed therapist. If you're feeling like you're holding the weight of the world, this book will speak to your soul, offer needed resources, and invite you into the sacred work of healing.

KAYLA CRAIG, author of *To Light Their Way*

Aundi shows a way beyond "toughing it out" and "what doesn't kill you makes you stronger," and it's a gentle and self-compassionate approach. Ultimately, it's the way of Jesus, and Aundi is a wonderful guide into it.

CHUCK DeGROAT, PhD, LPC, professor of pastoral care and Christian spirituality, interim DMin director, Western Theological Seminary

Strong like Water beautifully acknowledges the courage that survival requires and offers practical tools to move from simply coping to gaining embodied strength. Over your own deep waters, Kolber's voice will rise as a wise and gentle guide, calling forth your inner strength and testifying to God's redeeming love.

CLARISSA MOLL, author of *Beyond the Darkness*

Strong Like Water is such a timely book as so many of us deal with the pressure of needing to be the "strong one" in one way or another. This book is an encouraging guide that will help you gracefully navigate the many experiences of life that call for strength.

MORGAN HARPER NICHOLS, artist and writ

Finding the Freedom, Safety &
Compassion to Move through Hard Things—
& Experience True Flourishing

STRONG
LIKE
WATER

AUNDI KOLBER MA LPC

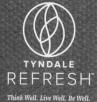

TYNDALE
REFRESH™

Think Well. Live Well. Be Well.

Visit Tyndale online at tyndale.com.

Visit Aundi at aundikolber.com.

Tyndale and Tyndale's quill logo are registered trademarks of Tyndale House Ministries. *Tyndale Refresh* and the Tyndale Refresh logo are trademarks of Tyndale House Ministries. Tyndale Refresh is a nonfiction imprint of Tyndale House Publishers, Carol Stream, Illinois.

Strong like Water: Finding the Freedom, Safety, and Compassion to Move through Hard Things—and Experience True Flourishing

Cover designed by Eva M. Winters

Published in association with Don Gates of the literary agency The Gates Group;
www.the-gates-group.com.

For information about special discounts for bulk purchases, please contact Tyndale House Publishers at csresponse@tyndale.com, or call 1-855-277-9400.

The case examples in this book are fictional composites based on the author's professional interactions with hundreds of clients over the years. All names are invented, and any resemblance between these fictional characters and real people is coincidental.

Library of Congress Cataloging-in-Publication Data

A catalog record for this book is available from the Library of Congress.

ISBN 978-1-4964-5471-3

Printed in the United States of America

29	28	27	26	25	24	23
7	6	5	4	3	2	1

For my mom—thank you for passing me your Hungarian fire.

For Jude, Tia, and Brendan—the loves of my life.

And for survivors everywhere:
may your healing come.

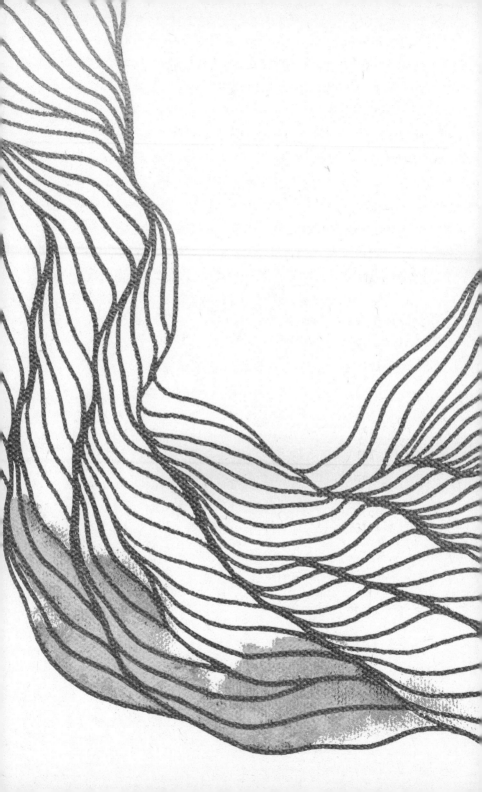

CONTENTS

WHAT IF THE

TRUEST STRENGTH IS AS

EXPANSIVE AS THE TIDE;

THE FIERCE & GENTLE

ELEMENTS DANCING

TOGETHER AS ONE?

INTRODUCTION

STRENGTH IN THE WAVES

Water: voice of grief,
Cry of love,
In the flowing tear . . .
Blessed be water,
Our first mother.

JOHN O'DONOHUE, *TO BLESS THE SPACE BETWEEN US*

THE WAVES OF THE MIGHTY PACIFIC OCEAN crashed in front of me; the sparkle of the water and the intensity of the shore break were almost hypnotizing. I buried my toes in the sand, which was speckled with rocks and black dust, as I took in the majestic view. I never tired of the ocean and came here often—mostly, just to be near it; to be regulated by the rhythms of the waves (though I didn't have words for that yet). I wanted to feel immersed in something much bigger and more powerful than myself.

The chaos of the ocean mirrored the tumult I felt inside. I'd graduated from college a few months before, but frankly, my life felt as if it were falling apart. Actually, it's fair to say that it was. I had called off an engagement and quit my first professional job within the span of a week. (For the record, I don't regret either of those decisions, but this certainly wasn't how I'd pictured my post-college life.) What I didn't realize was that, in addition to all those disappointments, I was still carrying around the effects of a childhood full of complex trauma that I hadn't begun to unpack. Its presence affected me every day.

I was only twenty-two, but sitting by this oceanside, I felt much older; worn. *Is life always supposed to feel this hard?* After a few decades of pushing myself at all costs to achieve and tying myself into pretzels for everyone around me—honestly, I didn't know who I was anymore.

Even more honestly? I was not completely sure I ever had.

Others told me I was the strong one, the spiritual one, the wise one, the responsible one, the good kid, the girl who would get things done. There was a part of me that liked these labels. And there was some truth to them—there was a ferocity as strong as the rushing tide that coursed through me. Many of these traits had been hardwired in me as a way to survive the tumultuous and at times traumatic household I'd grown up in, but my family's dysfunction had begun generations before. I carried my ancestors' pain as well as their strength: I was the daughter of a refugee who'd escaped in the back of an ambulance from a war-torn country when she was only four. I was the granddaughter of a man who'd survived a childhood of poverty by eating leftover corn from pigs and who had the audacity to flee Hungary with his family when the only other choice would have been to join the oppressor. I was the great-granddaughter of a Croatian woman so tenaciously determined to live that she'd fended off thieves with just her fists. These were the stories that had been passed on to me, and this was the fire and fierceness that ran through me.

And yet this strength had come at great cost, not only to my ancestors, but also to me. Kids aren't meant to hold adult problems or adult pain. Kids aren't meant to grow up when they're still small. Many of the qualities that folks affirmed about me were the result of living in and through trauma. I had never known anything different from the family I'd grown up in. What most people didn't see was how much it cost me to have so little support and to feel as if I was always on my own. To feel that the world was constantly on my shoulders; that I had to remain tough, responsible, and put together no matter what—it was a heavy burden to bear.

And so, like I'd done for much of my childhood, I let myself feel pain in one of the few places that it felt safe to do so—here, near the water. This was where I saw a glimpse of who I truly was. This was where I felt the Spirit of God. This was where I could find at least a glimmer of the peace for which I'd been looking; this was where God whispered that I was loved in such a gentle voice that I almost missed it. This was where I understood Jesus' words, "My yoke is easy and my burden is light" (Matthew 11:30). This was where I could sink into these words from the psalmist: "Be at rest once more, O my soul" (Psalm 116:7). This was one of the few places my body could fully exhale.

And finally, finally, she did. My body settled.

I wonder whether you've ever felt alone and weighed down by the burden of needing to be "the strong one"? Maybe you've found identity in your armor—your tenacity, your ability to survive. After all, it seems to be the thing people like best about you. Maybe you've tried to let others know how much you're hurting, but it's always ended either in your being misunderstood or experiencing heartbreak. So now when your heart is tender, you shame yourself or find a way to suck it up again; you've decided that vulnerability just isn't worth it. Sometimes it might seem like being unemotive—pretending and suppressing what you truly feel or need—is the only way you'll actually be loved at all. After all, it can feel as if society constantly berates you with these messages:

> No pain, no gain. Pain makes people strong.
> Well, at least you're going to learn an important lesson.
> Stop complaining; it could be worse.
> When the going gets tough, the tough get going.

Everything happens for a reason.
God doesn't give you more than you can handle.
Just pray about it.

Now, let it be said—there are elements of truth in those statements. When the going gets tough, the tough *do* get going. Faith and prayer *are* great resources to get through difficult experiences. Certainly, sometimes there is no other way to survive than to white-knuckle our way through life when circumstances require it.

And yet. When the idea that "what doesn't kill you makes you stronger" plays out in real life, we see that it just doesn't hold up. What doesn't kill us can actually make us isolated, traumatized, and deeply harmed if we don't receive the support we need as we go through it. We've internalized these platitudes and, as a consequence, we feel exhausted, burned-out, and disconnected from our truest selves. These phrases may come from well-intentioned sources, but unfortunately, they're only keeping us stuck—pretending; suppressing; believing the lie that *strength*, and ultimately wholeness, looks only like denying ourselves at every turn.

Is there a different way? What if emotional health doesn't *always* look like being "the strong one"? What if sometimes it means stepping back and letting ourselves receive or grieve or feel? What if it's not just facing hard things—though that matters—but *also* knowing our limits? What if it's loving others, but *also letting* ourselves be loved? What if the truest strength is as expansive as the tide; the fierce and gentle elements dancing together as one? What if this strength has the flexibility to be both soft and bold; to both nourish and protect—because it is rooted in a foundation of love rather than fear?

What could life be like if you were strong like water?

———————

At thirty-eight, sixteen years after I last watched waves pound on that familiar Pacific beach, I return.

So much has happened since I was last here. Within months of that long-ago afternoon at the ocean, I moved to Denver, where I soon met my husband, found my vocation, had two kids, and began hours of therapy and millions of tiny healing moments, all to piece together the fragments of my story that trauma had shattered. The first step had been letting myself be nourished as I learned what it meant to be truly strong. Not in the way I was used to—the strong that had required me to be something I wasn't; to pretend and suppress and ache. Not strong like the world often measures it—through brute toughness and forced smiles. Nope, this was different because God had begun teaching me to be strong like Him.

He taught me what it was like to receive and feel and grieve and savor and lean in and lean out and be fully alive— to be strong and flexible like water.

I sit in almost the exact same spot on the beach as I did when I was younger. I dig my toes into the black-speckled sand. I gaze at nearly the same view. But the experience is different because *I* am different. Not because I am perfectly healed. Not because I have all the answers. Not because I am now somehow impervious to pain. God is teaching me that no matter where I am in the process of healing, I am worthy of receiving love, compassion, care, and support. I finally realize that experiencing moments of both courage and tenderness is part of my journey.

Now I know what it's like to feel safe in my body. Now I know in the deepest parts of myself that I'm beloved by the God of the universe. Now I know how to find the people who make me feel like myself. Now I can honor the generational stories that helped shape my family. Now I know it's okay—beautiful, really—to feel my emotions. Now I know how to move through pain, rather than suppress or be toppled by it. Now I know what it's like to feel a solid sense of myself rather than constantly react to fear or trauma.

Now I know what it's like to be strong like water; to gather in the aching parts of my story and support them with compassion and hope. Now I know, and I can never not know again.

———

Reader, to gain that inner steadiness, you may need to unlearn some of what you've internalized about strength. You may begin to recognize that some of the ways pain and trauma have imprinted stories in your body must be examined with curiosity and compassion so you can come to the truer story: You can put down your heavy, ill-fitting armor now because you're already so loved.

To begin this work in part 1, we'll look at the high cost of living from *situational strength*; the kind of strong that may outwardly appear to carry you through stressful situations unscathed but that leaves you both anxious and high-strung as well as numb and exhausted. We'll discuss why this type of strength is worthy of honoring but ultimately isn't sustainable. (To make these concepts more accessible, I include client stories, all of which are fictional composites drawn from hundreds of professional interactions.) As we continue, we'll unpack a concept I call the *flow of strength*, which pictures the various forms of strength we embody. We'll also explore the many ways your nervous system and experiences of safety or unsafety shape you. We will consider how to utilize what I've come to call *compassionate resourcing* as a way to internalize glimpses of goodness, connection, love, and safety. All of this work will empower you to access an expansive, strong-like-water strength: from lifesaving to life-giving, ebbing and flowing in a way that is right for you.

In part 2, we'll focus on various compassionate resources that will support you and help you cultivate a more holistic, *integrated strength*. At the end of each chapter, you'll find various exercises to engage in at your own pace. It's my hope that, through this plethora of resources, you can experientially access the work of becoming strong like water.

If you've read my book *Try Softer*, it's my hope that in these pages you'll be able to take some of the lessons on being gentle and attentive with yourself further. If you haven't read it, don't worry—I have written *Strong like Water* in such a way that it should be accessible to every reader.

Dear one, the work ahead will be challenging at times, but I pray you will feel held and equipped as you learn to embody this more expansive view of strength. As you read, please keep in mind that much of this work is both bidirectional and parallel. That is, you may find that you circle around and through an idea, taking it as far as it can go, and still find that you'd like to come back to it later. Simultaneously, you may learn about another concept that you are able to quickly and aptly apply to your life. What's most important is that you have permission to make yourself at home in these pages. Although I believe the framework I've created will be beneficial as it's laid out, if you find you need to skip, adapt, or return to certain parts at a later time, I encourage you to do whatever will honor the pace of your story and body.

Additionally, I do my best to present my work through a trauma-informed lens, which means that even when we are focusing on concepts that foster growth, it's important that you honor your capacity. The experiences of your body matter, and I don't want you to push yourself beyond your limit in the moment. This will help ensure that the growth you experience is real and can ultimately be integrated in your body.

Please be aware that this book is not intended to diagnose mental health conditions or substitute for the important work of counseling. While I've done my best to present information in a way that feels accessible outside of the counseling room, you may need to work through some parts of your story with a licensed therapist.[1] This is completely okay. There is no shame in needing additional support—in fact, even noticing when this is true is quite brave. As a therapist and a trauma survivor myself, *I honor that the story you hold in your body is particular to you.* What is not traumatizing or overwhelming for someone else might be *for you.*

Dear one, I'm sorry you've experienced events that required you to survive rather than live. I'm sorry you've often felt alone and unseen. I'm sorry you've had to be so strong. And I'm sorry that you've never felt safe to be gentle with the parts of yourself that have needed tenderness so badly. I consider the work ahead of us to be sacred ground, and as I write this, I'm praying that this book will be a resource in the story of restoration God is weaving in your life.

I know that you may have experienced unthinkable trauma and/or violation. Before we go any further, I want to thank you for being here. I honor the courage required simply to show up to this page. Or maybe you are coming to these pages looking for affirmation that the hundreds of tiny cuts of pain you've experienced throughout your life are valid. I thank you, too, for being here. Maybe this sense of being alone or unsupported in your pain began in your childhood, or maybe it developed later in life—either way, it matters. Regardless of the story your body holds, I believe you are invited to a different, more expansive way of viewing healing, wholeness, and possibly—*especially*—strength.

God's posture toward any fragmented, hurting parts of yourself is one of compassion. May you embrace this good news as we begin our journey together.

PART 1

EMBODIED WISDOM: THE FLOW OF STRENGTH

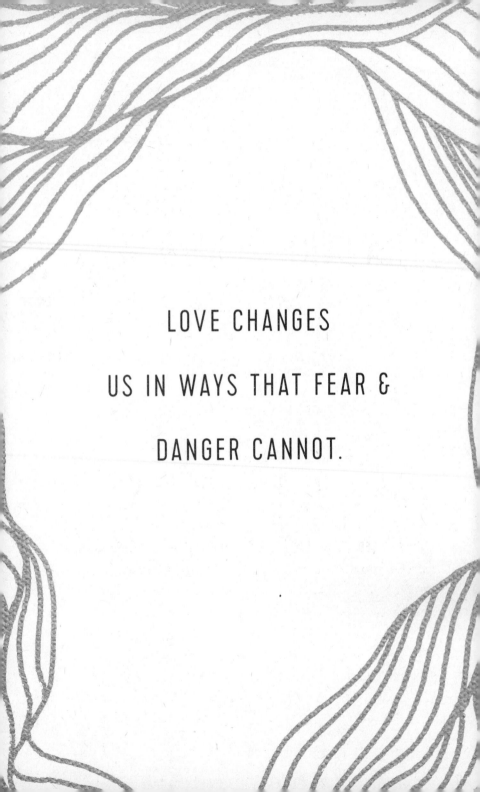

LOVE CHANGES

US IN WAYS THAT FEAR &

DANGER CANNOT.

CHAPTER 1

THE COST OF BEING (A CERTAIN KIND OF) STRONG

Trauma decontextualized in a person looks like personality.
Trauma decontextualized in a family looks like family
traits. Trauma in a people looks like culture.

RESMAA MENAKEM

"I'M SO TIRED OF BRACING MYSELF, AUNDI," Tiffany told me as she settled into the couch in my office. "I never know when my mom is going to blow up because I set a boundary or simply expressed myself."

The weekend before, Tiffany had been at a big family get-together where she'd tried to share a small sliver of her actual feelings with her mom.

"Oh, don't be so dramatic, Tiffany," her mom scoffed. An awkward silence filled the room.

Tiffany felt herself turning bright red from the shame of a humiliation that was both terrifying and familiar. This, she had told me many times, is what kept her feeling like she had to bottle everything up.

After telling me about this embarrassing experience, Tiffany continued. "People have always told me I'm so strong, but I'm tired of having to look like I have it all together—especially when it comes to my family." Her father had died of an overdose about two years before, and this had been the catalyst for huge upheaval in Tiffany's life. Not only was Tiffany grieving her father, but she was also beginning to realize how much her childhood had affected her. Memories of the many years she'd experienced verbal and emotional abuse from her parents seemed to float up overnight.[1] Her relationship with them had been strained, though she hadn't been quite sure why. Now she realized that the chaotic dynamic of their relationship had forced Tiffany to grow up in ways she hadn't been ready for.

And after her father's death, her relationship with her mom was even worse. One of the main problems? Tiffany's mom wanted her daughter to act as if nothing at all had happened. The more Tiffany stuffed her feelings, the happier her mother was.

Tiffany released a heavy sigh before continuing. "I mean, why do we have to pretend? The visit with my mom last weekend actually began fairly well. But when I started to tell her how important therapy has become for me so I can process everything I've been through these last two years, she cut me off. My mom wants us to white-knuckle and not show any grief, but doesn't she realize how much courage it takes to deal with so many difficult memories? Isn't that strong too?" Tiffany wondered out loud.

The truth is, it was. Tiffany and I had been doing work together for about six months, and I'd been moved by her progress. After making sure she had the stability to process some of her past, she was able to begin letting herself feel supported and giving voice to some of her deepest pain.

"She told me . . . she told me I'm weak for needing therapy," Tiffany whispered as the tears began to fall.

I sat in my chair across from Tiffany, heart racing. I wished I didn't hear something like this so often. But this wasn't the first time someone told me how they'd been shamed for trying to heal, and unfortunately it wouldn't be the last.

Tiffany had internalized a false narrative that had first bloomed in the earliest years of her childhood and then was upheld by her parents' rigid and at times punitive religious beliefs. They often told her—couching it in spiritual language—that if she was suffering, it was her own fault. If she felt alone, it was her own fault. If she burned out, it was her own fault. If she didn't have the tools to cope, it was her own fault. Essentially, Tiffany had come to believe and work from the story that everything hard in her life was her own fault. If she'd just been stronger, complained less, and been more faithful, things wouldn't have been so bad.

Maybe the way her father emotionally, verbally, and psychologically abused her wouldn't even have happened.

Maybe her mom would have done something to stop him.

Maybe her father's death from an overdose wouldn't still haunt her.

Maybe.

Tiffany was stuck. In order to maintain that connection with her family—and, she assumed, with God—she had to pretend, bypass, and find a way through no matter what, even if it was profoundly harmful. She felt deep shame and confusion for feeling so hurt; on the other hand, she couldn't see what she might have done differently. She needed her family. She needed to be a *good* Christian.

What other option did she have but to push through, suppress her pain, and do whatever was required to survive?

THE FLOW OF STRENGTH

From birth, we all are wired to need our caregivers, no matter the cost. Psychiatrist and trauma specialist Gabor Maté says it best: "People have two needs: attachment and authenticity. When authenticity threatens attachment, attachment trumps authenticity."[2] God designed us to instinctively know in our bodies that we need the care of others. And if we don't get adequate support—especially in our childhood years—we take whatever we can get so we can survive. We are as adaptive as the situation requires.

As I worked with Tiffany, she began to realize that she had not felt authentic safety as a child. Due to their own complex histories, her parents had been ill-equipped to provide one form of nurturing that is vital to human flourishing: co-regulation. Caregivers provide this when they recognize and respond to their children's distress or pain with empathy and attunement,[3] something Tiffany's mom and dad had largely failed to do. In encountering a co-regulating presence, children experience what Dr. Daniel Siegel calls "feeling felt."[4] When this happens, on a neurobiological level children have an embodied sense that they are not alone, that they are seen, that they have value, and that somehow things will move toward resolution.[5] These experiences of co-regulation and "feeling felt" become the platform of safety from which we most healthfully show up in the world. Ideally, we begin to learn these co-regulation skills as kiddos so that as adults we intuitively know how to engage them with others, particularly our own children if we have them.

But Tiffany's connection with her parents wasn't based on attunement and care—but rather was dependent on her *acting* the way they demanded. Tiffany was great at appearing okay, even when she wasn't; she had to trade her authenticity for belonging.[6] In the absence of true connection with those closest to her, she learned to look good on the outside but didn't actually feel safe on the inside. She learned to disconnect from all the verbal, emotional, and psychological abuse—and the gnawing sense that one mis-step would mean she would have nothing and no one. She demonstrated a tremendous will to survive in the face of deprivation.

It was through my work with trauma survivors like Tiffany that I began to reimagine how we conceptualize strength. Just as water can change from a gas, to a solid, to a rushing river or a gently flowing stream—so too has God imbued our bod-ies with this ability to adapt; this strength. And so I began to think: *What if all the ways we are designed to survive should*

THE FLOW OF STRENGTH

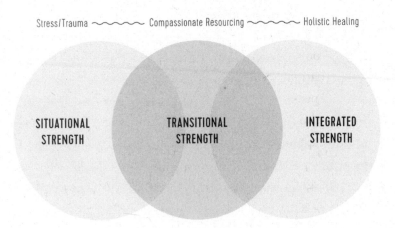

Stress/Trauma 〜〜〜 Compassionate Resourcing 〜〜〜 Holistic Healing

SITUATIONAL
STRENGTH

TRANSITIONAL
STRENGTH

INTEGRATED
STRENGTH

Though different types of strength are required in different situations,
compassionate resourcing (safety and support) is the current that moves us along the
flow of strength toward a more holistic and sustainable way to be in the world.

never be viewed as sources of shame but rather of honor? And what if strength is *also* found in all that is required to heal?

In other words, what if our innate ability to survive distressing, overwhelming, or traumatic experience *is* strength, but so are tenderness, compassion, feeling our feelings, and learning to rest? What if it's not a question of either/or but instead both/and? This, my dear reader, is what brought me to conceptualize the flow of strength.

The flow of strength idea is meant to help us visualize that, like water, our response to challenging circumstances is meant to be fluid. The more supported and safe we feel, the more we heal and grow, and the more flexible we will become. Like a skilled sailor, we learn to adjust to changing seas. At various times and in particular situations, different types of strength will be needed. This is completely normal. And as we'll discuss—important.

When our body doesn't experience a certain level of safety—be it physical, emotional, or spiritual—we will need situational strength to make it through. As we experience support, care, attunement, connection, and compassion, our bodies will naturally and intuitively begin to flow into an expanded strength, allowing us to live and act from the truest parts of ourselves. Even after we've experienced some integrated strength, the reality is that we may need to rely on our situational strength again at times—this doesn't mean we are bad or failing. Like water, we *flow*. We adapt, we flex, we use what we need in that moment. Having to access situational strength is simply information our body is giving us about our level of safety. At every point in this cycle, our bodies are working to keep us safe and alive—and this deserves to be recognized for the strength that it is.

I want to say this as clearly as possible: Our work here is not about a finish line. You may be tempted to picture situational strength, transitional strength, and integrated strength as categories on a scorecard—almost as if the more check marks you have in the integrated strength column, the more valuable you are. I know this may be challenging in a culture that is so focused on achievement, but I invite you to let go of this framework. Situational and transitional strength are *also* good gifts.

Many of us are unaware that we aren't flowing into these expanded areas of strength; rather, we are living only from situational strength, even when we are no longer in danger. It makes sense—our bodies haven't felt safe enough to believe there are other ways to be strong. We'll continue to unpack the wisdom of these strengths as we move forward, but for now, may we begin by recognizing that the whole flow of strength has a place and deserves to be honored.

Situational strength

When Tiffany first came to see me, her life looked impressive. But it didn't feel that way to her. Instead, it felt like life-or-death; it felt like if she were to stop living from her habitual patterns—overfunctioning, overachieving, over-accommodating others, and pushing herself until she felt numb—all her worst fears might come true. She hadn't felt safety and support from her parents, and she'd never been given the resources to feel secure enough to express her feelings and needs. Cognitively she knew she was an adult now with different choices, but her body still felt as if she were trapped by the threats from her childhood.

When we operate from situational strength, it means our bodies have moved into a stress and/or trauma response to navigate or neutralize difficulty. Sometimes we are facing a real danger: Think of how quickly a person reacts if they see a venomous snake while on a hike. Before they even have a conscious thought, their body reacts by running to ensure not getting bit. Or consider the mother who uses almost superhuman strength to lift a vehicle off a small child. We might also lean into parts of our situational strength in our everyday life, like when we're navigating a breakup or a difficult interaction in the workplace.

In temporary, short spurts, situational strength is extremely helpful, necessary, and even protective. And when the crisis has passed—and our body registers that it is over—we are designed to integrate the memory into the bigger story of our experiences and sense of self. We are then able to learn from, reflect on, or even build on what we've lived through.

But what happens when the experiences that require people's situational strength don't end? What happens when the danger passes, but it doesn't *feel* over? What happens when every time they consider their experience, their bodies

A Brief Guide to Stress/Trauma Responses

STRESS/ TRAUMA RESPONSE	DESCRIPTION	PHYSICAL SIGNS
FIGHT[7]	Our nervous system has determined that some form of *aggression* will give us the best chance of survival.	Increased heart rate, flushed or pale skin, dilated pupils, quickened breath, irritability, locked jaw, tight fists, anger, thoughts of harm toward others or self
FLIGHT	Our nervous system has determined that *fleeing* a situation will give us the best chance of survival.	Increased heart rate, quickened breath, restlessness, inability to focus, desire to leave or hide, trapped or anxious feelings
FREEZE[8]	Like a deer caught in the headlights, our body is working to determine the best course of action, causing us to appear still and "frozen" on the outside. (This is a common response in situations where we feel trapped, such as in childhood trauma, interpersonal violence, and/or sexual violence.)	Physical sensations of feeling cold, numb, stuck; a sense of dread combined with a sense of anxiety; immobility or a sense that we can't move; a sense that everything is both too much and not enough
COLLAPSE/ SHUTDOWN	Our dorsal vagal complex has determined that our best chance of survival is to disconnect psychologically, physically, or emotionally.	Decreased heart rate; physical sensations of feeling cold, weak, incapable; thoughts of apathy, despair; a sense of too muchness
FAWN[9]	Though more research is needed, this is the most complex response our nervous system has, potentially spanning different autonomic states in order to appease or submit to a threat (overaccommodating, overfunctioning, people pleasing) to increase the chance of survival.	

begin to go into the stress or trauma response meant to help them survive? (See the chart on page 22 for a refresher on the various types of stress/trauma responses our bodies can have when they detect a level of real or perceived threat.)

If we live out of situational strength for too long—whether because the danger is still present or the trauma is so deep—our experiences will remain fragmented in our bodies and psyche. This means that even the good or helpful parts of these experiences aren't available for us to leverage when we need them. With situational strength, we see everything and interact with the world through survival mode. If you grew up in a home, environment, or system that consistently felt threatening, this may be true for you too. You find ways to be strong, but it often comes at the cost of never finding and being yourself, the person you were created to be.

One way to tell if you're operating out of situational strength is a persistent sense of feeling unsafe; that what you're experiencing is life-or-death and/or that you are completely and utterly alone. Remember, this sense is a signal—not an indicator that you are bad or deficient. Your body reacts in this way to protect you.

Yet it's also a cause for grief. Living with this constant sense of threat and feeling chronically unsafe creates an urgency in your body that causes you to bypass or unconsciously ignore good things (past and present) that happen in your life.[10] As a result, you are less likely to be positively impacted by the support and resources that you *do* have. Your body quickly and unconsciously decides that it cannot spare any energy to focus on goodness because diverting attention from the bad could endanger your survival. For example, the teacher who worked tirelessly for his students may not recognize his tenacity because he spent much of his childhood trying to prove that he was valuable. The young woman who lived through a traumatic childhood, including experiences of racism[11] and poverty, may be unable to see the courage it took just to survive her life as a Black woman. The ER doctor who did her job under significant duress during the COVID-19 pandemic may have such overwhelm, disturbance, and trauma stuck in her body that it has created a barrier to seeing the ways she did show up. The mother who experienced significant relational harm and neglect as a child but now gets on the floor to play with her kids and tucks them into bed every night may struggle to see all the ways she actually is connecting with her children and how much each small step of healing matters.

From the outside, each of these folks may seem to be exuding strength. And unquestionably, they do have a certain kind of strength, one that is worthy of profound honor for what it has cost them. But without addressing the trauma interwoven with their strength as well as the lack of safety and resources after their trauma, the parts of themselves that showed tremendous fortitude and allowed them to survive hardship will remain unavailable.[12]

When we rely on one or more of the behaviors outlined on pages 26–29 to appear strong, we may get stuck in thinking that situational strength *is* the end game. As Joan Halifax says:

> All too often our so-called strength comes from
> fear, not love; instead of having a strong back,
> many of us have a defended front shielding a
> weak spine. In other words, we walk around
> brittle and defensive, trying to conceal our lack
> of confidence.[13]

Though we can honor our need for situational strength, when we get stuck in this rigid thinking, we may miss the possibilities of wholeness. And as a result, we come to think that pain, shame, or fear is what makes us strong. Our strong-like-water work is to learn how to validate the reality that situational strength has its place but also allow ourselves to move toward something more expansive; a truer version of what God intended for us.

I want to pause here and make something clear for those of us who've lived much of our lives in situational strength: I'm not asking you to abandon that fierce, "strong one" part of yourself. In fact, riding the ebb and flow of strength doesn't mean you lose any piece of yourself at all. Instead, this work is ultimately about inviting you to become more, not less, of your God-given self.

Ways Situational Strength Could Present Itself

Note: The following list is not exhaustive, nor is it meant to diagnose. Instead, it's meant to help you see that situational strength can be helpful in some circumstances, but if it's the only way you operate, it can have a high cost.

POSSIBLE EXPRESSION	HOW IT MIGHT SOUND (THOUGHTS/STATEMENTS)	
HYPERVIGILANCE[14] It feels safest to track every potential danger.	What was that sound? Who was that person? Why are we doing this?	
EXCESSIVE ATTENTION TO DETAIL[15] It doesn't feel safe to leave any detail to chance.	Here's a spreadsheet of every single thing that may happen in the next five minutes.	
HYPERINDEPENDENCE OR HYPERDEPENDENCE[16] It feels safe only if we do it on our own because we don't expect anyone to be there for us. or It feels safest to lose ourselves in someone else because we don't trust ourselves.	I don't need anyone's help, ever. or I need you to do it; you probably know better anyway.	
TOXIC POSITIVITY[17] It doesn't feel safe to acknowledge reality because we don't feel we have the resources to handle it.	I'm sorry you broke your ankle. At least it's sunny! Chin up!	
SPIRITUAL BYPASSING[18] We aren't certain that God will meet us in our pain, so it feels safer to use the idea of faith or spirituality as a way to not feel what we're facing.	If I pray hard enough, my trauma [depression, pain, poverty, etc.] will go away.	
PROFOUND TENACITY[19] The idea of failure or something not happening feels like (or might actually be) a life-or-death situation.	There is literally nothing that can get in my way (even if it hurts me or someone else).	

HOW IT MIGHT HELP US	HOW IT MIGHT HURT US
Enables us to stay "ahead" of the threat	Less able to be present in the moment (because we are constantly scanning for danger)
Creates some sense of certainty amidst overwhelming chaos	Inability to dream and stay flexible to change, which could lead to missed opportunities
Hyperindependence can appear to fit the classic idea of strength: not needing anyone can create high levels of perceived success. Hyperdependence opens us up to the beautiful reality that none of us can do this human gig completely on our own. We need connection to survive and heal.	In hyperindependence, we lose the essential resources of connection and community; as a result, we are more likely to remain stuck in a trauma response in the future. In hyperdependence, we risk becoming disconnected from our God-given individuality. (It's as though we've outsourced our own internal navigation system.)
Allows functioning in the midst of traumatic or disturbing experiences or events	Disconnection from reality and from what is required to actually process the event and heal
Similar to toxic positivity, provides a brief reprieve when a traumatic or disturbing experience feels overwhelming to our nervous system	Disconnection from reality; trauma or disturbances can become stuck in our bodies
Allows us to complete incredibly daunting tasks in the face of potential danger	Treating everything as life-or-death is a physically unsustainable way to live.

POSSIBLE EXPRESSION	HOW IT MIGHT SOUND (THOUGHTS/STATEMENTS)	
HYPERRESPONSIBLE We care more about other people's problems than they do.	*Oh sure, even though you should be the one to explain why you were late, I'll do it for you.*	
SEEMINGLY UNFAZED BY PAIN It doesn't seem safe to feel connected to our body so we miss the cues for pain.	*Wait, when did I break my leg?*	
EXTRAORDINARILY ACCOMMODATING It is safest to navigate the real or potential threat of our discomfort by giving someone whatever they want.	*No, it's no problem to get up at 2 a.m. to get you an ice cream cone.*	
USING SARCASM TO BYPASS EMOTION[20] It is safer to make feelings into a joke.	*Of course your telling everyone how I embarrassed myself in front of my boss is hilarious!*	
HUNKERING DOWN AND/OR ISOLATING Connection and/or functioning feels too risky and unsafe to our systems.	*Everything and everyone feels like too much; it's better to be alone.*	
ANY ACTION THAT IS ROOTED IN SURVIVAL ENERGY BUT DOES NOT DISSIPATE ONCE THE THREAT HAS PASSED		

HOW IT MIGHT HELP US	HOW IT MIGHT HURT US
Allows us to function when our caregivers or other primary attachments in our lives were or are currently unable to manage themselves	In adult relationships, it keeps the other person in a cycle of dependence; constant panic and vigilance is unsustainable to our mind, body, and spirit.
Enables us to "soldier on," even when we are physically unwell	Missed opportunities to listen to our body and respond in the ways we need
Become extraordinary at anticipating and responding to the needs of others to avoid direct physical, verbal, or emotional harm	High risk of burnout, trauma, and abuse (because we are constantly misattuning or denying our own needs and limits)
Serves as a way to navigate a situation without being further harmed	Keeps us from being known and knowing others, resulting in isolation and blocked healing
Allows us to experience a certain level of protection from potential threat	Profound disconnection from the support we need to truly live

Please know that after all you've been through—how you've had to be strong to survive—I'm proud that you're still here. And I'm not naive enough to believe that there won't be seasons and situations in this life where you may need to adapt and be strong like that again. But I also want to acknowledge that you and I have often paid a high cost just to survive.

When we don't have the safety, support, or resources to experience the completeness we need, it matters. It matters to God. It matters to us. It matters to how we show up in the world.

After working with me in the therapy room, my client Tiffany finally began to recognize the great cost she bore by having to stuff her emotions to appear strong. Though she deeply desired to experience belonging, having to be inauthentic around her family actually created a barrier between them. She finally saw that without safe connection, the belonging she experienced with her family was a poor substitute for the love and intimacy she truly longed for. When she became more empowered and settled, Tiffany began to see glimmers of how her friends and coworkers saw her and maybe even how God sees her: brave and beloved. As Tiffany internalized this love, it became a launching pad for her to move more boldly into transitional strength.

Transitional strength

Henry grew up with his grandma because both of his parents had been killed in a car accident when he was a baby.

Though Henry's grandma was loving, her health issues kept her fairly unavailable to truly support or attune to Henry as he grew. Additionally, they lived near or below the poverty line, and Henry frequently experienced bullying throughout childhood. Because of this history, as an adult Henry cognitively knew he was loved but often struggled to treat himself that way, leading him to dismiss his own needs in many situations. In the corporate world, his drive was often rewarded with bonuses for his willingness to work long hours and push hard. But all that came crashing down when Henry was diagnosed with a chronic illness that turned his life upside down—he was literally unable to overwork. Now how would Henry prove he was lovable?

As we worked together in therapy, I began to see Henry learn how to pay compassionate attention to himself. His sense of self-hatred softened, and he learned that listening to his pain was actually quite brave. Once Henry recognized that the way he had ignored and suppressed his needs had been a type of strength that helped him survive, he began to feel a new sense of self-respect. Gradually, Henry developed skills and resources that helped him attune to his body and wounds, as well as to interact with them differently.

I call the middle space along our strong-like-water flow diagram *transitional strength*. This is the place where we begin to attend to the wounds and/or traumatized parts of ourselves with safety, resources, and support—but unprocessed pain may still exist. Transitional strength is a space of duality where we begin to truly acknowledge that two realities can exist at the same time. We can have pain but also joy. We can feel grief but also hope. We know we're moving toward this space when we can observe how we're feeling or what we've experienced, and though we may not be glad about it, we can respect its impact and reality.

We'll discuss the characteristics and signals of transitional strength at length later in the book; right now, it's important to know that the significance of transitional strength cannot be overstated. This is the ground from which we truly begin to have a choice about *how* we engage our story, our body, and our strength. Until we connect to transitional strength, we are essentially reacting on a neurobiological level to what's happening. But from transitional strength, we begin to have more influence about how we interact with ourselves, our world, others, and our Creator. Much of the work I write about in my book *Try Softer* chronicles this important, sacred ground of attending to ourselves with gentleness, attunement, and compassion. And truly, because we are human, finite, and imperfect, we will always have elements of transitional (as well as situational) strength in our lives.

Yet, as we are able, may we have eyes to see the invitation God gives us toward connection and fullness; toward an integrated strength.

Integrated strength

From a neurobiological standpoint, integration reflects the healthiest and most resilient way we can be in the world.[21]

Consider the story of Janessa, who first sought counseling because of her history of childhood neglect. Janessa leveraged transitional strength to become aware of where this childhood trauma affected her most in her present life and worked to build a toolbox of resources to attend to herself with self-compassion. Then she gave birth to her daughter. The birth itself was traumatic, with several complications, as well as prolonged labor that ended in an emergency C-section.

Just a few days after her baby's arrival, Janessa unexpectedly began to have panic attacks and terrifying thoughts, and she *knew*—in a way she would never have been aware of in the past—that the traumatic experience she had been through deserved care and tender attention. Rather than stay stuck in situational strength, ignoring the pain and pretending she was fine, Janessa was able to acknowledge and honor her reality and, ultimately, fully process the trauma in therapy. The birth trauma she experienced was still a part of her story, but it didn't define Janessa anymore. She had acted from a place of *integrated strength*. A few years later, after noticing a passion develop around advocating for other women in similar positions, Janessa decided to become a birth doula. Though several years ago this role would have been frightening, her own experience had shown Janessa that a solidness existed in her; a belief that she was extraordinarily brave. She wanted other women to know they were brave too.

When we attend to our boundaries, emotions, and trauma, we open ourselves to love in the form of safety, connection, and belonging. I believe that, fortunately, God has given us tools that allow us to be truly, holistically strong. Not the kind of strength that is sometimes weaponized to tell people to "get over it" nor the kind of strength that causes us to deny reality or the needs of our body. Rather, we can develop the kind of strength rooted in love, not fear. The kind God lovingly offers and models for us: strength like water. What a profound paradox this tends to be when we consider our truest strength; everywhere we look we assume that it is pain that makes people tough. But as the wise researcher and psychologist Allan Schore has noted, the resilience is in the *repair*—not the wounding.[22] Schore was speaking to the importance of parents repairing with their kiddos after pain or a relational rupture, but the point stands: The strength of resilience doesn't happen because of wounding but because of what happens *afterward*. When pain and trauma are met with the love and support needed to repair the wounding, we heal—and by the grace of God, we are able to hang on to everything we learned from that experience.

Thankfully we have a God who knows all about love. John 3:16 begins, "God so *loved* the world that he gave . . ." (emphasis mine). This is the root; the beginning and the end. Our God is love. He is a God of shalom, wholeness, and completeness. Jesus said, "I have come that they may have life, and have it to the full" (John 10:10). And yet we hold this potential in tension with God's compassion toward pain. This is the God who says about His stance toward the weak: "A bruised reed he will not break" (Isaiah 42:3). Reader, I invite you to sit with that for just a moment. We can honor that we are worthy of the dignity offered us at any point along the spectrum.

What is God's love like? What is the source from which we experience love? The apostle Paul describes it this way:

> Love is patient and kind. Love is never jealous. It does not brag or boast. It is not puffed up or big-headed. Love does not act in shameful ways, nor does it care only about itself. It is not hot-headed, nor does it keep track of wrongs done to it. Love is not happy with lies and injustice, but truth makes its heart glad. Love keeps walking even when carrying a heavy load. Love keeps trusting, never loses hope, and stands firm in hard times. The road of love has no end.
> 1 CORINTHIANS 13:4-8, FNV

Ultimately, our tethering to love, hope, and safety is what makes us truly strong, and they are clear indicators that we're moving along the flow of strength. In this space, we feel pain, but we are not swallowed by it. Love, hope, and safety allow us to leverage, risk, and face hard things from a place of resourcefulness that is unavailable to us in survival mode. You see, love changes us in ways that fear and danger cannot. It both softens and strengthens us.

This work is not about arriving anywhere, though certainly it will impact how we live. We hold this truth in tension with the reality that God gave us bodies with the capacity to survive difficult situations. In fact, because we have access to the source of love, we are better able to embody what love is truly like as we heal.

BECOMING STRONG LIKE WATER: A PLACE TO BEGIN

I can think of about a hundred places I'd like to invite you to explore as we take this journey of becoming strong, resilient, and more fully ourselves. But what I've learned is this: Before anything else, we need to build and strengthen our safety and resources.

I have seen this truth again and again with the clients I serve, as well as in my own recovery from complex childhood trauma. Thus, the following practices are foundational for helping the body recognize it is safe in the here and now.

GROUNDING RESOURCE

One resource I frequently teach to folks I work with *and* utilize in my own life is grounding.[23] Clinical psychologist and trauma expert Dr. Arielle Schwartz notes that grounding "refers to our ability to experience ourselves as embodied . . . to sense [our] body, feel [our] feet on the earth, and as a result calm [our] nervous system."[24] We engage our five senses to the extent that we are able to bring our body and awareness into the present. We do this because, God willing, the present moment is safe—or at least safer than the moments we are recalling when we feel flooded or overwhelmed.

Though there are many ways to practice grounding, one simple way is to engage the language of *noticing* as you use your different senses. You can do this practice anywhere, although if possible, it's especially helpful to get outside.

To begin, use this language with yourself as you actively seek out:

a. "I'm noticing [something I can see] _____."
b. "I'm noticing [something I can touch] _____."
c. "I'm noticing [something I can hear] _____."
d. "I'm noticing [something I can smell] _____."
e. "I'm noticing [something I can taste] _____."

I invite you to continue to use this practice until you begin to feel more regulated or for as long as it feels helpful. As always, if at any point this resource starts to make you feel further triggered or flooded, you can discontinue it.

CONTAINMENT RESOURCE

There are times it's not only appropriate but also *necessary* to create some internal space between ourselves and that which feels too disturbing or overwhelming to connect with. When this is the case, we can create a psychological "container" to help us create this space.[25] We don't use containment to suppress pain but instead to mindfully access it in a way that restores choice—we get to decide how we engage with it. Often trauma survivors have had little power in moments or experiences that were disturbing, so the hope is that practices like these can be a part of the repair.

1. In your mind's eye, consider an object or space that feels like it might be able to "hold" the disturbance you're experiencing. Please know you can be as creative with this as feels helpful. For example, I've had clients picture placing their overwhelm in a spaceship and launching it into the sky, putting their pain in a huge safe, or even picturing God's hands holding the disturbance for them.

2. After you have your "container" in your mind's eye, consider what feels disturbing or overwhelming as you scan your body from head to toe. (If this is your first time doing this practice, I recommend choosing something mildly disturbing/irritating to practice with.) As you consider your disturbance, picture a laser starting at your head and going all the way to your toes to locate where in your body you feel it. After you've located it in your body, take a moment to see if you can place this disturbance in your container. Know that you can take as long as you need to fully place the disturbance all the way into the container.

3. As you do this, your body is going to give you the best information as to whether your container is "strong" enough. If you begin to feel some relief after placing your disturbance in the container, this is a sign that the container is sufficient. However, if you don't experience relief, you may consider placing your original container into an additional container(s) to create more layers between you and the disturbance. For example, you could take a bank vault you imagined and then place that entire vault at the bottom of the ocean.

4. Finally, once you experience that sense of space, name your container. Take a moment and notice the space you feel and then create a name that helps convey what you're feeling.

As a reminder, if at any point this practice no longer feels helpful, I invite you to discontinue and/or utilize grounding instead. Generally speaking, the more triggered or activated you feel, the more likely it is that you will need several resources. In that case, you may wish to begin with grounding, contain whatever still feels disturbing, and then go back to grounding. As always, I invite you to tweak these resources to make them work for you. Finally, I encourage you to reach out to a licensed therapist if you need additional support.

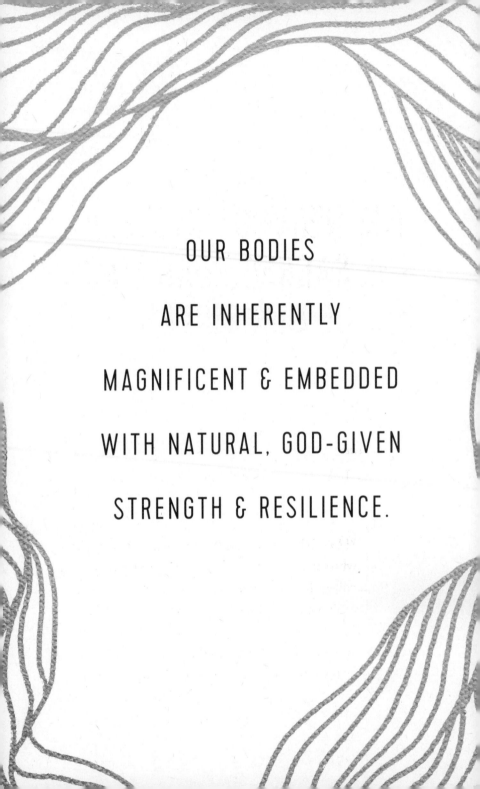

OUR BODIES

ARE INHERENTLY

MAGNIFICENT & EMBEDDED

WITH NATURAL, GOD-GIVEN

STRENGTH & RESILIENCE.

CHAPTER 2

THE NERVOUS SYSTEM: THE SACRED ROAD MAP OF OUR BODIES

There is a voice that doesn't use words. Listen.

RUMI, THIRTEENTH-CENTURY PERSIAN MYSTIC POET

I'M TWELVE YEARS OLD WITH KNOBBY KNEES and a big heart. My sister—who, in my mind, essentially hung the moon—is home from college for the weekend. Steph knows how much I love basketball; the way I play in pickup games every chance I can. Already I've learned to be scrappy and tenacious. She also knows how scared I become when my parents fight and my dad becomes terrifying. From her own experience, she understands the chaos my other siblings and I still face at home. I'm fairly sure she realizes that I will need to be fierce to survive these next few years.

"Aundi, come here. I have something to show you," Steph says.

We walk outside to our empty street. She looks at me and smiles, a gleam in her eye. She begins dribbling, first on her right side, then crossing over to her left, then through her legs.

"I've learned that dribbling is like dancing," she tells me as she bounces the ball. "You've got to have some rhythm. Here, let me show you a move."

My eyes light up. Steph plays a different position than I do, but she knows I will likely be a point guard, so she spends time teaching me specialized skills. It feels good to be cared about like this. As we begin to practice, I give all my body, breath, and focus to the moment.

Slow, slow, quick: I dribble.

Slow, slow, quick: This is the rhythm I learn for the crossover.

Over and over again we dribble the ball up and down the street. Every dribble feels a bit more natural.

"You're a warrior, sis!" Steph calls as I pick up speed.

The Oregon rain begins to fall, lightly at first and then in a downpour, but I don't mind. We practice for at least a few hours. I begin to feel like maybe I can be who she says I am.

I'm seventeen, and my crossover still serves me well. I've been the starting point guard on my high school's varsity team for four years. I play basketball like my life depends on it—maybe because in a sense it does. Some part of me knows that basketball might be my way out of the dysfunction, and I channel all my anger, sadness, and pain onto the court.

It's true that I love the game itself. I love how the ball feels in my hand. I love when the game is on the line and I get the chance to help the team win. I love knowing I left every single thing I have on the floor. But I also love feeling like I have some power. I play with such heart and tenacity; people ask what motivates me: "Where did you learn to play with so much *fire?*"

What they don't know is that with my family, I have to be ready for anything, that I feel helpless to the whims of the abuse at home. Yet deep inside me, pressure from the trauma, harm, and neglect has been creating magnificent diamonds of tenacity, ferocity, and passion, which feel as if they are wrapped in dynamite. If I can't let that fire explode at home, I'm sure going to bring it on the court. Having a place to feel capable and influential matters a whole lot.

Later, I'll joke with people that Jesus and basketball saved my life. What they don't always know is that it's actually true.

I'm twenty years old. I play college basketball and go to an excellent school. I've done it; I've moved away from home. But I'm plagued with a sense of confusion: I thought that once I left home, the trauma would leave too. It has changed in some ways, but it still haunts me. Now it shows up as a sadness that never leaves; an aching hole. Now it shows up as romantic relationships that hurt me and constant anxiety that I'm all at once too much and not enough for everyone I meet. I feel frozen.

Sure, my tenacity still shows up on the basketball court, but I wonder, *What good is my fierceness when it can't soothe the ache everywhere else?*

———

I'm thirty-five now. I feel as if I've lived whole lifetimes since college; I've done hard work and gained considerable compassion for my own story.

One afternoon I find I'm reflecting on my journey with basketball. I begin to consider those priceless moments with my sister, and tears fall rapidly. For so long, I couldn't think about memories of basketball without also activating a response from my childhood trauma; my heart beating wildly, a pit forming in my stomach, and a sense that I had to be brave or *else*. There was much goodness in those memories, but it was wrapped up in so much pain.

I've since learned that the situational strength I brought to basketball was essential for me in that time of my life; it allowed me to weather a traumatic childhood. Yet, because it was born out of a need to survive, that ferocity also felt disturbing to my body for many years because I had not yet fully processed the trauma connected to it.

I was afraid of my warrior self.

The thought of connecting to my fierceness—the fire that so many people had praised for so long—and bringing it to other parts of my life felt terrifying.

That's why in order to fully honor my whole story, I've had to learn to see how my body—in particular, my nervous system—had been helping me survive trauma. Because each time I felt safe, every time I felt threatened, every time I felt hope or joy or grief, my body had been helping me hold these experiences as best she could. But the wisdom of my body knew I needed to stay somewhat fragmented, or disintegrated, until she felt safe enough to feel it as a whole.

THE WISDOM OF THE WINDOW

Through my clients and my own life, I have come to learn the value of tuning in to the information our nervous system reveals about our experiences. In many ways, I liken this knowledge to a sacred road map. After all, only in learning to listen to and honor the signals from our bodies can we ultimately move toward healing, toward a more integrated strength.

Our bodies are inherently magnificent and embedded with natural, God-given strength and resilience. But after we experience unresolved difficulty, we may come to fear them and disconnect from them in any way we can. We do this because they are the holders of our wounds. Our bodies are the very location of our trauma. And if it's never been safe to feel our pain—if we've been shamed for naming it, or we've not been given support as we do so—it makes complete sense that rather than have compassion for ourselves, we would instead fear this part of our humanity.

A Brief Guide to Our Autonomic Nervous System (ANS)[1]

The ANS is the part of the nervous system that controls unconscious functions like breathing, heart rate, and visceral responses to threat. It is made up of two main parts:

- The sympathetic nervous system (SNS) helps us mobilize when we experience threat. Depending on the level of arousal we feel, we may go into fight, flight, or parts of fawn. This is often known as hyperarousal.

- The parasympathetic nervous system (PNS) has two main functions:
  - First, it enables our bodies to "rest and digest"— what we experience when we are calm, present, and/or when we're in our WOT. This is often compared to a brake because it allows us to slow down. This is a vital part of our experience as humans and the state in which

One of the most transformative concepts around our nervous systems that I teach my clients is that every person has a range of arousal in which they can feel their feelings or experience something in a way that is tolerable to *their bodies*. This range is called the window of tolerance (WOT),[2] a term coined by Dr. Dan Siegel and further strengthened by the work of Dr. Stephen Porges.[3] If you've read *Try Softer*, some of our discussion here may be review. However, the WOT is such a foundational topic to almost all healing and growth work that I am confident it will continue to serve you.

Ideally, we will spend the majority of our time inside or at least connected to our window of tolerance; this is the place from which we can deeply connect with others and practice curiosity, awareness, and even creativity. When we are inside our WOT, we have access to our full brain because our body isn't experiencing or perceiving overwhelming threat. By learning to incorporate, honor, and leverage our window of tolerance, we each have the potential to heal, grow, and move toward a more expansive strength.

When we are connected to but not fully inside of the WOT, we are experiencing what is sometimes known as a blended state.[4] We have one "foot"[5] firmly planted in the present, knowing we are safe and have choices and support we can lean on when needed. Our other "foot" is fixed in whatever mildly to highly distressing sensation, emotion, or memory we are facing. As a result, our brain and body are mostly online, but we may sense some level of threat activation. This is transitional strength; a location from which, with practice, we can observe ourselves and begin to have some choice.

But when we go outside our window—because our body detects or perceives a threat—we will typically go into a fight or flight response. If that doesn't resolve the threat,[6] our body may shift into a highly adaptive trauma response called the fawn response (which focuses on neutralizing a threat by either over-accommodating or ultimately submitting to a threat). Or finally, when our body senses that no other option will be helpful, we may go into a form of dissociation

we hope to spend the majority of time.

- The second part of the PNS is related to a less advanced part of our physiology known as the dorsal vagal complex. This is sometimes referred to as hypoarousal and is the part of our nervous system that becomes activated when our bodies perceive a threat so significant that, as a way to survive, we go into a freeze, collapse, dissociation, or parts of the fawn response.

Those of us with a history of unprocessed trauma may find that our bodies activate both our SNS and dorsal vagal at times when we are not experiencing a present threat. Instead, threats from the past are being reactivated in our bodies. In order to unlearn, move through, and ultimately heal from trauma or other emotional disturbances, learning to work with our nervous system is key.

ranging from the freeze response all the way down into collapse. In this state, we begin to go off-line; that is, much of the blood flow to the logical, decision-making part of our brain (our prefrontal cortex) is redirected to the lower, more survival-oriented parts of our brain. The *only* goal is survival.

The further we move outside our window, the more off-line our prefrontal cortex becomes. Yet, when we have the tools and awareness to support the way our bodies are wired, we can better help them respond in alignment with our values and who God designed us to be.

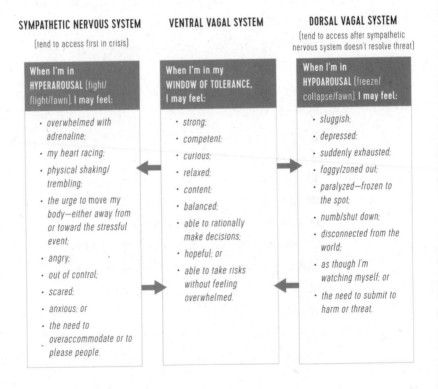

SYMPATHETIC NERVOUS SYSTEM
(tend to access first in crisis)

VENTRAL VAGAL SYSTEM

DORSAL VAGAL SYSTEM
(tend to access after sympathetic nervous system doesn't resolve threat)

When I'm in HYPERAROUSAL (fight/flight/fawn), **I may feel:**

- *overwhelmed with adrenaline;*
- *my heart racing;*
- *physical shaking/ trembling;*
- *the urge to move my body—either away from or toward the stressful event;*
- *angry;*
- *out of control;*
- *scared;*
- *anxious; or*
- *the need to overaccommodate or to please people.*

When I'm in my WINDOW OF TOLERANCE, I may feel:

- *strong;*
- *competent;*
- *curious;*
- *relaxed;*
- *content;*
- *balanced;*
- *able to rationally make decisions;*
- *hopeful; or*
- *able to take risks without feeling overwhelmed.*

When I'm in HYPOAROUSAL (freeze/collapse/fawn), **I may feel:**

- *sluggish;*
- *depressed;*
- *suddenly exhausted;*
- *foggy/zoned out;*
- *paralyzed—frozen to the spot;*
- *numb/shut down;*
- *disconnected from the world;*
- *as though I'm watching myself; or*
- *the need to submit to harm or threat.*

Show over tell

Thinking back to my basketball days, it is easy to tell someone how to dribble a ball or shoot a jump shot, but it's the lived experience that truly causes that knowledge to come alive.

It's the same with our brain and nervous system. We receive information from our nervous system through sensations, intuitive movement, and emotions. In addition, this system highly prioritizes the conceptual idea of show over tell—or, to put it another way, lived stories over statements of fact.

When we are trying to write a new story, we will have the best results when that narrative is rooted in an experiential process. The words we speak to ourselves and others always matter because they communicate some degree of truth or intention. However, if they are not grounded in something that *feels* true in our bodies, they won't stick. Or to put it another way, it's somewhat easy to tell ourselves we have value, but it's a whole different thing to experience a visceral connection as you speak those words, *knowing* they are true. This is why, throughout this book, I give you tools you can use to build awareness of your moment-to-moment personal experience. This is the framework that allows actual change to happen.

You might be reading this section and feel tempted to count yourself out. Maybe you don't feel like you've ever had the lived experience I'm describing; you've never felt loved, valuable, capable, or anything else. My dear reader, if this is you, I want you to know two things. First, I'm so sorry. I see you, and I honor your reality. And second, I have written this book with you in mind. I want to tell you that you haven't missed your chance on wholeness; as lovingly as I can, I ask you to be open to the work we'll do in the pages ahead—because I'm going to teach you how to keep your eyes out for these reparative experiences so that your body can experience them as true.

Discomfort versus harm

Tuning in to our nervous system allows us to draw the important distinction between discomfort and harm. We may be tempted to think of these words as synonyms, but our bodies actually experience them very differently. When we experience discomfort, we experience something that is challenging or hard, *but we remain connected to our window of tolerance*. Alternately, harm can be thought of more like an injury; moving far beyond discomfort and requiring us to tap into only survival energy. Neurobiologically, I would define harm as requiring us to go into a stress/trauma response (completely leaving our window of tolerance) to navigate it—typically without support for it to be processed through our bodies.[7]

As counterintuitive as it may seem, discomfort can be a holy thing. It's actually an important part of the way we grow.[8] We need to be able to tolerate some discomfort to engage the dance of being human; sometimes we make mistakes or harm others, and it's important that even though it's uncomfortable, we look to repair.

But whereas the fruit of discomfort is ultimately growth, the consequences of harm will create destruction. For example, consider a new runner who gradually paces their body as they build up their speed. It may not be easy to do this, but it is not creating an injury because of *the way* it's being done. This is what discomfort is like. But if you take that same runner and require them to ignore the information of their body and push far beyond their capacity, there is a high likelihood that it will cause this person physical harm. For many trauma survivors and others who have learned to disconnect from their bodies, it is quite normal to be like the second runner, routinely pushing themselves—both physically and emotionally—into harm without realizing it until it's too late. For example, if a person has learned to please other people (fawning) as a way to navigate an unsafe household, they may not be able to recognize when the way they are genuinely caring for others is beginning to personally harm them.

Now caring for and accommodating others are beautiful ways to love our neighbor as ourselves—when we actively choose them. But if the body automatically defaults to putting others before ourselves, *no matter the cost*, the action is rooted in a trauma response and can be harmful. Thus, when we begin to learn *in our own bodies* what it feels like to pass over the threshold from discomfort into harm (and remember, it's going to look different for each of us!), we will be empowered to better understand and connect with what we need to honor ourselves and act wisely.

The paradox of being human is that we need discomfort to grow; but it must occur at a pace and in a way that our bodies can tolerate. Without the crucial distinction in our bodies between discomfort and harm, we may unwittingly interpret anything that is uncomfortable as harm. In a beautifully redemptive way, as we come to honor our own bodies we are better equipped to "love our neighbor as ourselves" because we gain more capacity to attend to the ways we affect others too.

A flexible nervous system

Becoming flexible and adaptable is a key part of learning to become strong like water—and amazingly, God designed us to be both.

There isn't one right way to respond to everything. You may have heard the saying that when you are a hammer, everything looks like a nail. We can get "stuck" in a certain way of being. Take Theresa, for example. She grew up with an older brother who constantly bullied, berated, and even hit her. When she tried to tell her single dad, he basically rationalized it by telling her the bullying would make her "tough." As a result, Theresa's body adapted the best way it could: by learning to fight at the drop of a hat. Now, even when she's out with a group of friends and a goofy joke is made or someone looks at her in a way she perceives as aggressive, Theresa is right back there as her ten-year-old self, ready to defend herself. It's exhausting for Theresa and has been hard on her friendships too.

Given her background, Theresa's reaction makes a lot of sense. And yet, because Theresa hasn't yet had the safety and support needed to process her past trauma, her body reacts to *any* situation—safe or unsafe—in the way she had to in the past in order to survive.[9] This is an example of nervous system *inflexibility*. Her body is reacting with situational strength because it has kept Theresa alive.[10]

And yet, the invitation to be strong like water remains for Theresa—and for each of us. As we honor the information of our bodies and respond with compassionate care, our nervous system also responds by becoming more flexible and capable of responding accurately to the information in front of us.

We can also look to Jesus' life to see a model of nervous system flexibility. At the wedding in Cana, Jesus celebrated. (Can you imagine how fun that wedding would have been?) When people were hurting or afraid, He showed them compassion. When He saw that the Temple was being used in a way that harmed God's people, He became angry. When He observed that the most religious people had weaponized their faith to make it inaccessible to the most marginalized, He became stern. And when He saw how grief-stricken Mary and Martha were when their brother, Lazarus, died, He was moved, and He wept. Jesus' nervous system was flexible, adapting to the situation at hand and helping Him live authentically and intentionally.

And for us, just like Jesus, part of our work is to compassionately develop a healthy, flexible nervous system that is able to respond accurately and appropriately to various situations.[11]

CONNECTING THE WOT AND THE FLOW OF STRENGTH

In the same way that our bodies and nervous systems can shift toward the WOT/ventral vagal, so too can we shift from situational strength toward integrated strength. Consider Theresa's story above. Because of her experiences of being bullied by her older brother, her body learned to quickly and reflexively move into situational strength to ward off real or perceived threats. If you consider her experience through the lens of the WOT, we're conceptualizing that when she's in situational strength she is *outside* her WOT.

Several of Theresa's friends come alongside to offer help. Theresa admits she'd like to find a therapist, but it's been an overwhelming task. Her friends decide they will help her secure a trusted therapist who, along with the support of Theresa's friends, guides Theresa in unwinding the trauma from her body. It's slow work, but eventually Theresa feels safe enough to compassionately explore the idea that, though she was harmed by her brother in the past, the present moment does not hold danger.

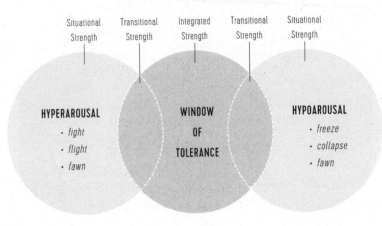

STRENGTH AND NEUROBIOLOGY

As Theresa begins to internalize the support offered to her, her intense fight response begins to fade; as it decreases, she increases her skill set of noticing what's happening in her body whenever she feels threatened. Now, Theresa has moved toward the edge of her window, beginning to flow out of situational strength and into transitional strength. Here she begins to feel she can *choose* how to react; she feels capable of working with and listening to her body.

And then, little by little, she learns to move toward the center of her window of tolerance. Hints of integrated strength start to shine through in Theresa's life as she learns to fully move through her grief and her anger. While she knows that her healing will be a lifelong journey, she has a new perspective on the world—and has the resources she needs to navigate it well.

As you read this, I invite you to notice this vital element: It is of the utmost importance that we heed the signals from our nervous system. Among other things, these cues will tell us if our body is in or outside its window of tolerance. As we've discussed, the extent to which we feel connected to a sense of safety will be the extent to which our body will be able to come back into our window of tolerance and ultimately will inform the way we move along the flow of strength.

Importantly, the more complicated or chronic the trauma that has us trapped in situational strength, the more time we may spend in transitional strength, building resources that can compassionately support the disturbance our bodies are holding. And yet, dear reader, as slow as this movement toward integrated strength may be, not a moment of your attention and care devoted to this work is lost—even if the journey ahead is long. For each of those moments communicates to your body that you are worthy of compassion and care.

BECOMING STRONG LIKE WATER

As we learn what it means to hold the tension between our desire for growth and our need for safety and resourcing, how do we begin to live from a place of deeper integration?

One idea I teach many of my clients and the thousands of folks I've interacted with over social media is this: We must begin with *honoring*—respecting the inherent dignity and value that we and our fellow image bearers share. We honor our stories, our pain, and the actual flesh-and-blood realities we live with. There is no bypassing reality, and there is no bypassing the bodies that have carried us in and through this reality. This is where we *must* begin. Not because all truth is found here, but because without our whole selves there can be no true healing. When we experience difficulty through the lens of respect and dignity, we are more likely to be able to move through what comes our way.

Most healing occurs as we move toward wholeness and integration, which gives us access to fullness of life. Sometimes I think about this when I read Jesus' words that He came that we may "have life, and have it to the *full*" (John 10:10, emphasis mine). How can we honor our pain and yet know we are created for fullness? I recognize that pat answers won't do the job here, and that's okay.

As I write this, we are twenty months into a once-in-a-century pandemic we didn't see coming. Back when it began, when we had just a shadow of how hard it would be, I wrote these words: "This feels hard, because it is hard."[12]

The death, the loss of freedom, the fear, the sickness, the anger, the polarization, the scarcity, the pain. It feels hard because it is and has been hard. Most of us have had to tap into our situational strength in some way during this season. The idea of "safety" has felt far off and almost laughable for many people. Those who had experienced a certain level of healing before the pandemic may have found themselves either triggered again or retraumatized. Folks who were already carrying the burden of chronic trauma, poverty, racism, discrimination, or other hardships may have felt those experiences intensified or worsened. Certainly, we do not want to make our home inside grief, but let us be clear: Unless we make room for the reality of our entire human experience, grief will insist on taking over the whole house.

But as we are able, God invites us to see what *is* so we can unlearn all the untrue narratives, keep our eyes open for safety and goodness, and enter the deeper and truer story. Dear ones, we don't have to pretend that simply existing doesn't hurt sometimes. It does and it has. Instead, without bypassing this reality, we are invited to move toward the resources that will allow us to soften into hope.

A PRAYER FOR HONORING

As you feel comfortable, find a safe space and settle into these words. You might even put your hand on your heart and close your eyes between sentences:

God, here in this moment, empower me to honor everything that arises in my body, mind, and soul today; even if it means I have to return to it at another time.

Creator of all things, remind me that in honoring my experiences, You help me affirm dignity to the parts of myself that have at times felt stripped of it.

God, help me know that my desire for safety and connection is valid. In Your wisdom You designed me to need both.

But as I'm able, grant me the ability to open up to the possibilities
of healing and newness while staying connected to the reality of Your
love.[13]

As you proceed in your strong-like-water work, I invite you to utilize this prayer whenever it feels like it may be supportive. I encourage you to remember that, paradoxically, the honoring and softening of our pain taps into our deeper strength—and you are never alone as you do so.

HONORING YOUR CONTAINER

An embodied experience of pain and trauma requires an embodied experience of repair and healing. In this journey, it matters that you give your body tangible language to help support yourself as you move through the world differently.

One important term is *capacity*. Somatic psychology proposes that each person has an emotional/psychological/physical capacity that can be thought of as a physiological container.[14] One way to picture this capacity is to think of yourself as a cup that can hold a certain amount of liquid. As soon as a person meets or exceeds their capacity, they will go outside their window of tolerance, and their stress, trauma responses, and/or situational strength will be activated.

Imagine two glasses. One is about one-fifth full, and the other is about four-fifths full. Obviously, the first glass can receive more before it will begin to overflow. This is a picture of what it means to say one person has more bandwidth or capacity than another person. This is not a judgment on the value or dignity of either person; it's just reality. People's capacities may differ based on genetics, story, history, and current circumstances. And for some people, much of their capacity is being used by seen and unseen variables: past trauma, disabilities, stress, racism, loneliness, mental health issues, chronic illness, difficult relationships, financial worries, discrimination, and more. Each of these elements is valid and affects the body, mind, and spirit in ways that are not merely abstract—they impact people's functioning. A glass can hold only so much and so can we.

GETTING TO KNOW YOUR CONTAINER

Let's begin with a practice that aims to simply build awareness around how much you may be holding in your life, spirit, body, and mind right now.

First, give yourself permission to name any challenges, pain, or trauma you are holding by simply writing them down (please feel free to be as detailed or as broad as needed). Examples include a history of trauma, the pandemic, a strong inner critic, a demanding job, a lack of a job, or experiences of racism or discrimination.

Once you've written down all that you are holding, take a moment to notice what you sense in your body. If possible, consider what you might say to a close friend who is holding what you are. If it feels like a resource, consider how God might feel toward you and what you're holding. What do you notice in your body as you consider this?

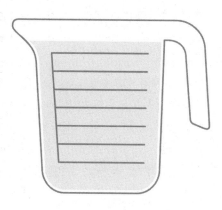

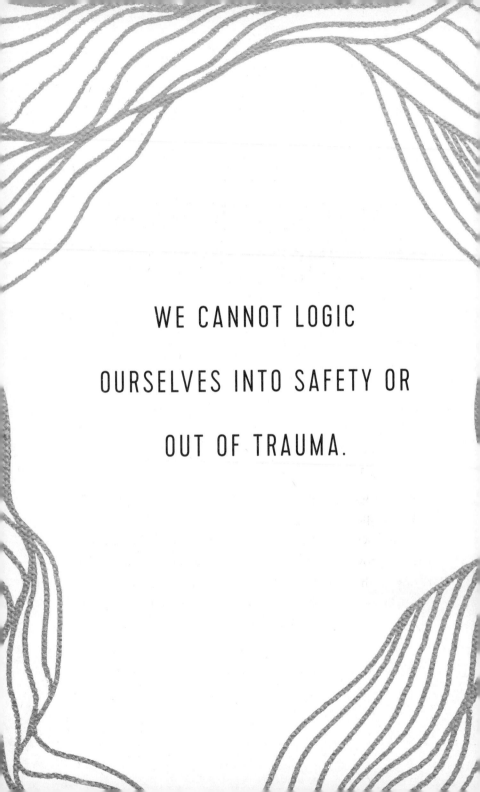

WE CANNOT LOGIC

OURSELVES INTO SAFETY OR

OUT OF TRAUMA.

CHAPTER 3

SAFETY IS THE MAGIC INGREDIENT

Feeling safe is the treatment, and creating safety is the work.

DR. STEPHEN PORGES

"WHAT WAS THAT?" Melina asked after my office door rattled a bit. Though we were midconversation, her body seemed to freeze up.

Our discussion stopped. From the outside, Melina looked like the proverbial deer caught in the headlights. But in the context of her story, I knew there was much more going on: At various times in her life, a door rattling had meant great threat. Between her father's explosive anger and the sexual violation she experienced from a "trusted" family friend, Melina's body was wired to react at just about any sound.

She knew it wasn't rational, but now whenever a door shut, Melina's whole body became taut with fear. When she heard that sound in the therapy room, I observed her first become hyperaware. Then, almost as quickly, her eyes seemed to glaze over, and I sensed she was no longer fully present. When this happened, we had to address it immediately and effectively, or her body would continue to move into shutdown. During our time together, Melina and I worked hard to build both an environment of trust and an understanding of Melina's unique nervous system. I invited her to check the door at the beginning of each session, and we practiced grounding exercises to make sure she was in the present moment.

But on this day, the door rattled, and nothing helped. This happened occasionally—even after trying her grounding practices, Melina would tell me she was feeling particularly fuzzy and not herself. Now in an attempt to engage more of her senses and provide additional support, I asked if she'd be willing to smell an essential oil as a way to help root her in the present. Melina said yes, but I didn't check with her about which one would be best. I began unscrewing the lid for my lemon essential oil, but as soon as the scent reached her, Melina's entire demeanor changed—and not for the better. She turned away from me with her lip trembling. "I—I don't want to smell that," she said, voice breaking. "Can we . . . can we please try something else?"

My heart sank. In my haste to help Melina feel safe, I hadn't asked her if this particular smell was okay with her—and to the surprise of us both, the smell had triggered something terrifying for her body. By all accounts my office was physically and emotionally safe, but the lemon scent made it so that Melina didn't *experience* it that way. Though pleasant smells have the potential to soothe, certain ones can be extremely triggering since they have a direct line to our amygdala, where much of our trauma is encoded.[1] Instead of helping, the lemon scent further activated a disturbing memory from the past that Melina's body was now experiencing as though it were the *present*.[2]

Realizing my mistake, I gathered myself so I could stay attuned to Melina as I put the essential oil back in my drawer. I slowed my breathing—making sure I was firmly connected to my window of tolerance—and gave Melina a heartfelt apology for not asking if that smell was okay for her. As I apologized and my regulated nervous system connected with hers, Melina's body language shifted. I could see some relief in her face, telling me that our momentary rupture had been repaired.

While we had made some progress, it was clear in that moment that Melina's sense of threat was still activated, so I offered her another scent to keep grounding her body in the present moment. We continued helping her regulate until she was firmly back in her window of tolerance. We could then resume our sacred work toward healing.

THE SCIENCE OF SURVIVAL

When we go through something difficult, it is so very human of us to want to do whatever we can to get through it as quickly as possible. We just want to move on, to not be affected by whatever caused us pain in the past. But the truth is, there is no bypassing the information from our bodies. We cannot "logic" ourselves into safety or out of trauma. Telling our bodies that we're safe and *feeling* safe are two very different things.

During my work with Melina, she came to see that her body was giving her vital information about the way she was experiencing the world—and my office in particular—on a subconscious level. This occurs mainly through the body's "autonomic surveillance"[3] system of neuroception, a term coined by Dr. Stephen Porges. Essentially, we are wired with neuroception to help us survive: It is constantly assessing our environment, ourselves, and the way we interact with others for cues of either safety or threat.[4] When neuroception pathways do not detect danger, and we have the appropriate amount of internal and external connection,[5] we *feel* safe (sometimes this is called "felt safety"). We feel calm and connected to our bodies, others, and our environment as we are solidly in our window of tolerance; we are curious, compassionate, and creative.[6]

When our neuroception picks up a potential threat, however, we automatically shift into various states of protection, depending on the level of danger our body detects. We do whatever we need to do (whether that means going into fight/flight, fawning, freezing, or a complete shutdown) to get through the situation. In Melina's case, as soon as she heard the door rattle in my office, her body detected the

WORKING TO BUILD FELT SAFETY

Our experience of felt safety, according to therapist Deb Dana, is the result of everything that occurs inside us, outside us, and between us. It's important to remember that our experience of safety is perceived and not necessarily literal. This is why, even when the world is tumultuous or hard, it's possible for us to work toward felt safety with ourselves and others.

**RELATIONAL
EXPERIENCE OF SAFETY**

*I feel safe &
regulated with others.*

FELT SAFETY

*In this moment, I feel
fully safe.*

**INTERNAL
EXPERIENCE OF SAFETY**

*I feel safe &
regulated with
myself.*

**EXTERNAL
EXPERIENCE OF SAFETY**

*I feel safe &
regulated in my
environment.*

potential danger; before she could even have a cognitive thought, her body worked to protect her. Though eventually Melina was able to grieve that her body had carried such a heavy burden of hyperawareness, over time in therapy she also came to recognize the amazing way her body had shown up for her all these years.

Just as incredible, we can leverage this key system of wiring to work for us. When we learn to become aware of our neuroception, we gain *perception* on the reality of our circumstance and can act accordingly.[7] This is what is happening when we move into transitional strength. Instead of situational strength and/or our trauma responses running the show without our knowledge, perception helps us work *with* our body to bring it back into our window of tolerance.[8] Additionally, with care and attention, our body gains capacity to more accurately assess the risk we are facing in the here and now rather than being overly influenced by experiences from the past.[9] And as we can do that, we have increased capacity to move along the spectrum of strength, partnering with our transitional strength and potentially integrated strength too.

WITHOUT SAFETY, WE SUFFER

Reader, whether you consider yourself a survivor of trauma or simply want to gain more understanding of your body, consider this important idea: Your body is constantly shifting and adapting to help keep you safe. I cannot overstate the foundational experiences of safety and supportive connections to our healing journey. As Dr. Bessel van der Kolk states, "Being able to feel safe with other people defines mental health; safe connections are fundamental to meaningful and satisfying lives."[10] Importantly, it is safety—*not pushing through*—that does the heavy lifting to bring us into our WOT and ultimately toward integration. In fact, when our body picks up cues of danger, it is "biologically unavailable"[11] to access our social engagement system (WOT), the area where the most advanced ways of handling difficulty reside. Author, therapist, and racialized trauma specialist Resmaa Menakem writes, "Bodies—white, Black, and otherwise—don't care about what's rational, possible, or true. They just want to experience safety."[12] It's a prerequisite to just about everything else. Quite literally, we cannot regulate our emotions, learn, or think rationally unless we feel a certain degree of safety. To restore that safety, our bodies move into what is meant to be a temporary stress response. And sometimes it works. Sometimes we run from the attacker or we jump out of the way of a moving vehicle or we avoid the place that gives us the creeps. But for many folks, efforts to find safety don't work; we become traumatized—and we suffer for it.

Our bodies testify to this reality. In my own experience and for clients like Melina, there has been a high cost to chronic experiences of feeling unsafe. A lot of this cost comes in the underfunctioning of our *vagal brake*. This is the part of our vagus nerve that is utilized when we are in our window of tolerance, and it is responsible for tempering our stress response to be proportionate to the circumstances.[13]

Our vagal brake works with neuroception to assess whether our body has enough safety to successfully navigate a situation—that is, whether or not we can stay in our window of tolerance (also called ventral vagal complex). And it partners with other systems in our body to keep us there; for example, modulating our heart rate to stay below about seventy-two beats per minute.[14] When our body needs energy to play catch or go on a walk, our vagal brake allows

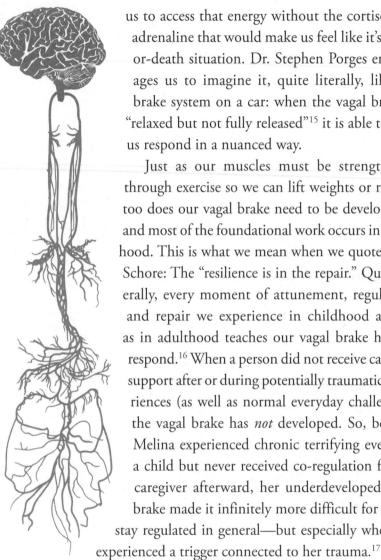

us to access that energy without the cortisol and adrenaline that would make us feel like it's a life-or-death situation. Dr. Stephen Porges encourages us to imagine it, quite literally, like the brake system on a car: when the vagal brake is "relaxed but not fully released"[15] it is able to help us respond in a nuanced way.

Just as our muscles must be strengthened through exercise so we can lift weights or run, so too does our vagal brake need to be developed—and most of the foundational work occurs in childhood. This is what we mean when we quote Allan Schore: The "resilience is in the repair." Quite literally, every moment of attunement, regulation, and repair we experience in childhood as well as in adulthood teaches our vagal brake how to respond.[16] When a person did not receive care and support after or during potentially traumatic experiences (as well as normal everyday challenges), the vagal brake has *not* developed. So, because Melina experienced chronic terrifying events as a child but never received co-regulation from a caregiver afterward, her underdeveloped vagal brake made it infinitely more difficult for her to stay regulated in general—but especially when she experienced a trigger connected to her trauma.[17]

Reader, the implications cannot be overstated. To return to the car example, bodies with underdeveloped vagal brakes are like automobiles with super-charged acceleration but no brakes. Once the gas is pushed, our bodies may skyrocket out of our WOT and into hyperarousal even at the smallest of scares (which is how Melina reacted in my office). And because there are no brakes, we may not be able to slow down until we crash into a ditch (hypoarousal).

If our vagal brake is almost non-existent, then *everything* has the potential to be an emergency, and we must stay vigilant or disconnected in order to stay highly protected against possible threats. No wonder we need to be ready to be situationally strong all the time! In the past, everything *was* an emergency. Our window of tolerance shrank, and we formed patterns of protection just to survive.[19]

NO TIME FOR GOODNESS

By all accounts, my client Georgia was impressive. She'd graduated with honors from a prestigious college, and then after successfully launching her own business, she became a highly sought-after

A Brief Guide to the Vagus Nerve[18]

The vagus nerve is the longest cranial nerve in the body, running from the brain into the face and ears, then down to major organs in the chest and abdomen, including the heart, lungs, intestines, and stomach.

One section of the vagus nerve is what enables us to stay in our window of tolerance. In polyvagal theory, this area is referred to as the ventral vagal complex. It enables us to use our social engagement system, which facilitates deep connection and co-regulation. The more we learn to co-regulate and self-regulate, the stronger our vagal brake will be, which helps us inhibit our stress response (when appropriate).

The far less advanced section of the vagus nerve is called the dorsal vagal complex. When our body decides the threat is too great, it may plunge us into frozenness, disconnection, dissociation, and/or collapse as an attempt to neutralize the situation.

consultant in her field. Georgia seemed to have a happy marriage and loved her four kids dearly.

After going over a bit of Georgia's history at our initial session, I still wasn't completely clear on what she hoped to work on in therapy.

"Georgia, I'm so glad you're here. I know we discussed a bit of your history with anxiety over the phone, but I wonder if you'd be comfortable sharing a little more with me about what you're looking to accomplish in our time together?" I asked as our initial get-to-know-you small talk petered out.

"Well, this is going to sound strange; that's why I didn't write it on my intake," she said. "Basically, everything in my life is going well—at least it looks that way from the outside. But I feel like I can't enjoy it. No matter what I do, I feel anxious or amped up or filled with dread. It's like a cycle that never goes away. It feels like Whac-A-Mole; as soon as I deal with one worst-case scenario, three more pop up. It's like I can see everything that could go wrong all the time. It's exhausting."

Georgia paused. "I guess I thought by now I would be able to enjoy my life."

We began our work by exploring Georgia's background, and she told me about one of her favorite pastimes as a child. She'd spent hours looking for beautiful, interesting rocks for her collection; obsessed with the process, Georgia spent most of her extra time reading about geology. She loved everything about rocks—from their shapes to their colors.

But when she was nine, Georgia's parents told her they were divorcing. At that point, Georgia left her collection behind. She developed an intense fear of being unprepared—because, in her mind, if she had just been more aware of what was going on back then, she would have seen the divorce coming. If she hadn't been so enamored with and distracted by her rock collection, she would have realized that her family was disintegrating.

So at age eleven, after a brutal custody battle that effectively took her away from her mother, Georgia vowed to herself that she would never again be unprepared. She would never let pain find her like this again. It was the only way she wouldn't get hurt.

This became Georgia's mantra as she went through life—be prepared for anything all the time. And in many ways it had served her well. Nothing ever surprised her. But the hypervigilance cost Georgia so much.

No amount of success, beauty, kindness, or connection ever seemed to make a lasting difference. All the ways she'd succeeded in business, the ways her husband loved her, the ways her kids wanted to connect with her, all the people who cared about her and respected her—she couldn't really feel it. She didn't resonate with them because her body had learned they weren't helpful. Sure, they were nice, but would they keep her from devastating pain? They only served as a distraction—beautiful rocks that she no longer had time for.

Feeling unsafe shapes the brain

The human brain and body are phenomenal in numerous ways. One example is our innate plasticity. This ability to shift, change, and grow is a beautiful gift that our Creator gave us, facilitating many important processes in our body. Plasticity allows us to do more than I can possibly describe here, but it is especially pertinent in our strong-like-water work. Plasticity helps us heal from trauma and other types of pain. Additionally, plasticity is what has actually allowed us to adapt and survive chronically disturbing, overwhelming, or traumatic experiences in the first place.

Trauma is not (and never was) a gift. But our bodies' ability to adapt so that we can survive? *That's* the gift; that's grace. And it gives every one of us a reason to hope.

Though we maintain plasticity throughout our lives, our brains are especially malleable in childhood. New neural pathways are constantly being created wherever blood flows.[20] When we respond to cues in our environment, blood flow (or energy) is instantaneously directed toward the response that our body deems appropriate for the situation. It's almost as if a new road is being paved in our brain. As the old adage (known as Hebb's axiom) goes: Neurons that fire together wire together—what we pay attention to quite literally changes our brain. And before we know it, we form new templates of how we experience the world and what we believe about it. If the blood flow and energy of a child's brain is constantly directed toward managing a threat—for example, in Georgia's case, being caught unaware by the oncoming tragedy of her parents' divorce—rather than connection, it will have a lasting effect. Certainly, it's important for us to acknowledge that every human has a leaning toward what is known as a "negativity bias,"[21] which causes us to focus on bad news or criticism more than on what is good. It's thought that this bias is influenced by our drive for survival. Yet it's also vital to name that, for trauma survivors in particular, this negativity bias is ramped up significantly, which impacts the shaping and firing of a person's brain and nervous system.

This is what happened in Georgia's case. The many instances of bravery, resilience, and strength she experienced through the years didn't seem to stick. This wasn't because she wasn't "choosing" to experience goodness and growth; instead, her body had unconsciously decided it was *not safe* to savor them. When Georgia began to understand how hard her body had worked just to keep her alive during the chaos that followed her family's breakup, she understood why it was still so difficult to truly experience good things.

This is why I grieve when I hear people say they "had to become an adult" before their time. This is why hearing that you're "so mature" doesn't always feel like a compliment. Our bodies are *designed* to receive a certain level of care and support, and it's traumatic when we don't.

What experiences can begin lessening our overall capacity? The times we weren't asked if we were okay. The times no one sat with us as we cried. The times no one was there when we ached. The times it felt too scary to stay connected to our own body. The times we had to figure it out on our own because our parents/caregivers weren't okay. The times addiction sucked the life out of our homes; the times spiritual abuse shaped the narrative, leaving us mistreated. It all adds up. Just as plants can't grow in soil stripped of nutrients and nourishment, neither can we.

Sure, when someone says a child is acting "mature" or even "more adult than many of the adults I know!" it sounds as if they're describing good behavior, but it can also mean that the child has learned to "trade in patterns of connection for ones of protection," as therapist Deb Dana so aptly describes.[22] If you were shamed every time you expressed an emotion, you eventually may have learned to deny and suppress that emotion (hypoarousal). In the short term, this may have kept you from being shamed, but in the long term, you missed out on beautiful opportunities for connection and co-regulation with others. And that leaves a mark—on your body, on your soul, on your brain.

THE SAFETY IS IN THE REPAIR

The paradox of this work is that in order to heal and move toward integrated strength, a level of safety and connection are *prerequisites*. With clients like Georgia and so many others who struggle to connect with the positive experiences in their stories, we must ask: How do we communicate goodness—even safety—to our bodies when we have lived through experiences that have been legitimately unsafe? How is that possible?

Embodied repair is the answer. Reader, this is why I care deeply about what I've come to call *compassionate resourcing*. Psychologist and author Dr. Arielle Schwartz writes that "a resource is anything that communicates safety to our bodies in the present."[23] Thus, compassionate resourcing is learning to have a posture of *coming alongside* and *remaining responsive to* the parts of ourselves and our stories that *do not yet* feel safe. Then, at the pace and in the ways we are able, we begin to offer experiences, connections, and moments to ourselves that *do* communicate safety. Each of these tiny (and not so tiny!) moments of repair help to expand our window of tolerance, as well as strengthen that all-important vagal brake.

For Georgia, we started small: We made sure to honor her limits as she learned to be with goodness, little by little. We did this first by helping her notice her experience during moments and events that were neutral; for example, doing grounding exercises and recognizing the relief she felt when she used containment (as practiced in chapter 1) to give herself some internal space from an overwhelming feeling. We gently built on this by helping her intentionally notice when something worked out, when people in her life were consistent, when beauty presented itself. It was slow work, but little by little Georgia was able to mindfully strengthen her vagal brake and increase tolerance for experiencing beauty, hope, and love. The good parts of her life began to hold as much weight as the trauma she had endured. Once her capacity grew, we were able to truly work through past traumas and find healing.

As always, it's important to acknowledge that sometimes it's best to begin this work with a therapist or a trusted other. But my dear reader, the effort is worth it: As our own sense of safety grows, we learn to be able to stay in the present moment from a place of regulation—and from this place, we can choose what we need to move forward and face hard things.

THE GOD WHO ORIENTS US TO LOVE

Trauma, pain, sin, and brokenness can be so disorienting. When we've been harmed—or even when we've been the ones who've harmed others—it can be difficult to find strong footing in who we are and who we are becoming. It can be hard to know where to begin to search for the safety we so desperately need to heal.

In the Garden, after Adam and Eve missed the mark by making a choice that didn't align with God's heart for them, "the man and his wife hid themselves from the presence of the LORD God" (Genesis 3:8, ESV). It doesn't take much imagination to picture the shame and disorientation Adam and Eve must have been feeling.

Yet as my friend and fellow therapist Chuck DeGroat points out, God *still turned toward them*[24] when He asked Adam a vital question: "Where are you?" (Genesis 3:9). In a sense, Adam and Eve had tried to disconnect from God's love, but God's love didn't disconnect from them. God came for them, even in their sin. Chuck writes, "God makes an incarnational move. God moves toward them, searches them out, and when God finds them they are clothed by the Divine Seamstress. God's movement toward them signifies an indelible message—I am your God. I will be with you. I will not abandon you."[25]

The question "Where are you?" was one God could have answered Himself. After all, He is omniscient; He always knew where they were. A part of me wonders if He posed it to help Adam (and Eve) internalize that question—so that they would, in turn, ask it of themselves as well. God is not only the Redeemer who ultimately saves us but also the Midwife who helps us birth a new way to be in the world. One action God takes to love us is to orient us, not only to time and space, but also to God's own self.

I love how Cole Arthur Riley writes that this is a story of "a God who kneels and makes clothes out of animal skin" for Adam and Eve.[26] What a tender and full picture of God's love for us. If we orient ourselves to the good, the true, the beautiful—to Love itself—we can begin to learn how to carry that around with us everywhere we go.

As a parent, I've invested much time helping my kiddos pay attention to their bodies so they learn to use the restroom, notice their hunger cues, and listen to their emotions. The language we use in our house is something like this: "Tia, Jude—can you please check in with your body?"

Every time I gently ask my kids to check in with themselves, I am not only helping them learn in real time, but I am also giving them a framework for how they might do this in the future: I am *orienting* them toward a way to be in the world. God willing, someday my kids will check in with their bodies without any prompting from me. But until then, I model it for them, helping them create strong neurological pathways and frameworks for how to be in the world.

I can't help but think this is a bit of what God was doing with Adam and Eve. He was modeling, creating templates, and ultimately helping them find a way through the consequences of their actions. God was orienting them to His own self and in doing so, teaching them what it meant to find solid ground again.

When we remember God's with-ness, when we remember how God has shown up for us, when we have eyes to see the goodness around us even through the smallest details of nature, we can find glimmers of hope. He is always making a way for us to reconnect, to experience even the smallest glimpses of safety. Just as the Israelites learned to raise their Ebenezers ("stones of help"; see 1 Samuel 7:7-12) to the many ways God had been faithful, we, too, can orient ourselves to what is true now, to the many ways we've already been loved.

Let me be clear: The lesson isn't to force ourselves to feel something when we don't—that would instead potentially be called spiritual bypassing or toxic positivity. Rather, we discover that when we work to orient our wounded parts to a new reality, we create truer connection and change. We are simply present to what is, especially when we are now physically, emotionally, and spiritually safe.

And so we ask: God, as we are able, may our lives be oriented toward hope.

BECOMING STRONG LIKE WATER: BUILDING SAFETY

Because we know that safety is a foundational part of what it means to be strong like water, I invite you to engage the practices below as you feel able to continue to build a tether to safety.

ORIENTING AND VAGAL NERVE STIMULATION

In this practice, we are going to work on communicating felt safety to your body by orienting it to the space you are in. We will then add a practice to stimulate your vagus nerve to help you continue developing that important vagal brake.[27]

I invite you to settle into a seated position on the floor or in a chair. If needed, you can practice grounding beforehand to give you a better chance to connect to your WOT.

Now, take a moment and look around the room. Notice the space. Notice the door. Notice the details of the furniture. Notice how old you are. Notice details in the space that help you know how old you are. As you do, see if you can allow your breath to settle into a rhythmic pace. Do what you can to avoid forcing your breathing and simply allow it instead.

Now, look over your left shoulder (doing so stimulates your vagus nerve) and find a fixed point to look at for up to thirty seconds. As you do, notice if you sigh, blink, or yawn—this is a sign that your body is moving toward your ventral vagal state (WOT). If you notice this, take a moment to let yourself sink into any sense of calm or groundedness you are feeling.

Repeat this same process on your right side. After you experience a sense of groundedness while doing so, come back to center and again orient yourself to the room.

As you're able, notice if you feel more calm, clear, regulated, or if any other supportive sensation has become stronger.

BREATH AS A RESOURCE

You may want to consider integrating the following Scripture verses regarding safety into the practice mentioned above or anytime it seems helpful.

As you practice with these breath prayers, I encourage you to inhale through the nose and exhale through your mouth. If you are finding your body is leaning toward anxiety, you may also consider doubling the length of your exhale; this communicates a sense of safety to our nervous system.

Psalm 9:9:
Inhale: The LORD is a refuge for the oppressed,
Exhale: A stronghold in times of trouble.

Psalm 32:7, BSB:
Inhale: You are my hiding place.
Exhale: You protect me from trouble; You surround me with songs of deliverance.

Psalm 116:2, NLT:
Inhale: Because he bends down to listen,
Exhale: I will pray as long as I have breath!

Psalm 91:1-2:

Inhale: Whoever dwells in the shelter of the Most High will rest in the shadow of the Almighty.

Exhale: I will say of the LORD, "He is my refuge and my fortress, my God, in whom I trust."

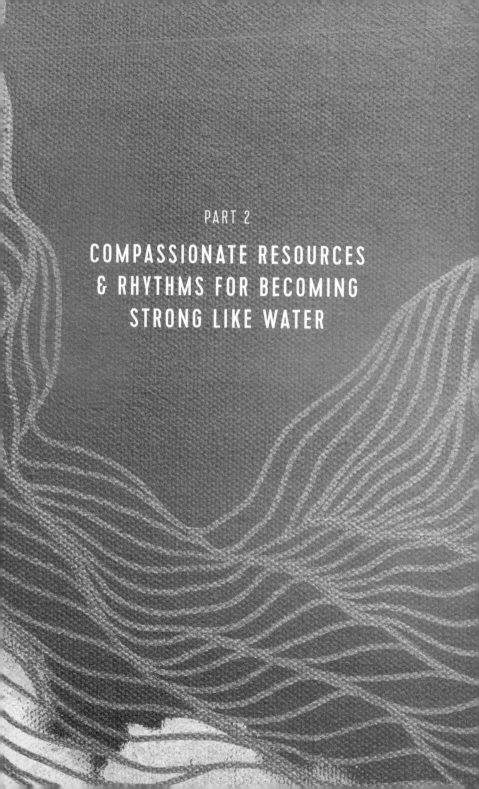

PART 2

COMPASSIONATE RESOURCES & RHYTHMS FOR BECOMING STRONG LIKE WATER

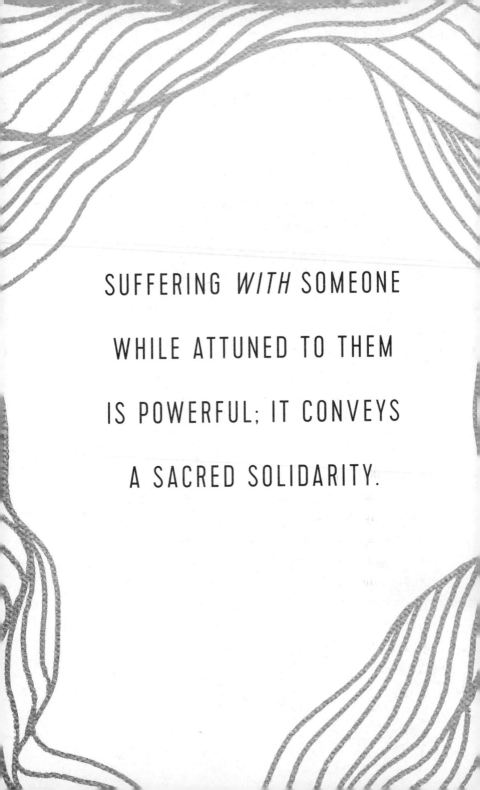

SUFFERING *WITH* SOMEONE

WHILE ATTUNED TO THEM

IS POWERFUL; IT CONVEYS

A SACRED SOLIDARITY.

CHAPTER 4

STRENGTH WITH CONNECTION

May there be an undoing of aloneness.

DR. HILLARY McBRIDE

ONE MORNING, just a few months after Brendan and I were married, I sat holding a cup of lukewarm coffee on the pink couch in my parents' living room. My eyes were red from crying. Just days before, this old but beautiful house had been sold. Cognitively, I knew selling the house I'd been raised in had been the right decision. My parents were in the middle of a contentious divorce, and this place was much too large and expensive—not to mention too much work—for my mom to keep on her own.

But this was one more change—many of them painful—

happening in a short period of time. In retrospect, I can see that this season marked the undoing of most of my family. When my parents split up, most of our family's belongings had been sold, and my dad had decided he no longer wanted to have a relationship with any of his children.

It was a lot. And it was painful.

Together Brendan and I had flown back to Oregon for a friend's wedding and then driven to the coast to see my family and say goodbye. I don't mean to dramatize saying goodbye to a house—houses are bought and sold all the time—but this particular property had witnessed much pain, heartache, and loss. My sadness at seeing it sold was not so much about the house itself, but more about all that it represented. Because of my story, there was just so much grief. I was grieving the loss of my dad, my parents' marriage, and the sense of family (fractured though it was). I was also mourning all the losses that accompanied my childhood. I felt grief about what didn't happen then, grief about what did happen, and grief about what couldn't happen. In my soul, that morning felt sort of like a funeral.

After a few decades of being a certain kind of "strong," I found it deeply disorienting to have so many wounds exposed at once. My situational strength couldn't keep up. I was still quite young, but I felt much older than my years. I had no idea how to navigate what was happening in our family, and though I'd started graduate school to become a counselor, I found it challenging to connect what I was experiencing with anything I'd learned in my program.

As I sat on the couch that morning—heavy with emotion—Brendan joined me, holding my hand. Already in the short time we'd been married he'd done this often; listening as I tried to make sense of the way my family was disintegrating, laughing with me when I couldn't cry anymore—reminding me that he was with me and wouldn't leave. Then he gently asked if I'd like him to take pictures of the house so I could be sure I'd remember it.

"Yes," I said, between sniffles. Gradually Brendan made his way around the house and then finally back to the room where I sat. As he stepped back to snap a picture of our long living room, he also captured me on the couch. It's not a glamorous photo in the slightest: me, sitting with my hair in a messy bun, my heart in pieces. I remember feeling ashamed that I felt so needy, so cracked open, grieving what felt like my entire world falling apart. All the situational strength I had acquired in the twenty-four years I lived in that house was beginning to show its edges; it was unable to keep me going.

Only now when I look at that picture and reflect on that painful memory can I see something else alongside the grief: Brendan's love and care for me, tethering me to hope and safety amidst the trauma of loss. After living through a few decades of unresolved and chronic relational, emotional, and psychological trauma, this was no small thing. Brendan was one of the first people whom my body, mind, and soul felt truly safe with. And not only that, something in me was beginning to learn that even when we faced challenges, we would make it through together. I had no language for it then, this liminal space—a space where I began to receive the support and resources I needed to be "with" pain. I've since come to call it *transitional strength.*

It's important to acknowledge that accessing transitional strength didn't cause the hardship and pain of that season to go away. Brendan's love and the therapeutic work I had already done to process my story did not save me from all the grief that lay ahead. It could not heal the trauma and abuse I'd suffered in that house. And in no way did it shorten the years of therapy and work needed for me to move toward a more integrated strength, to more fully inhabit my healing. But if ever there was a time I needed an embodied knowing that someone was in my corner, it was then. Brendan's presence communicated to my body that I wasn't alone. I could begin to tap into the belief that even here—in the middle of some of the hardest hard I had experienced—God's love was still for me too.

Other people had loved and supported me before this moment, but this experience was markedly different.[1] For the first time in my life, with Brendan, I no longer felt I had to trade my "authenticity for belonging"; I was truly safe. I no longer lived with my family, and the parent who had caused me the most harm no longer wanted to know me. The grief sat right next to the promise of healing.

But even if only for a moment, I was able to allow goodness, safety, and connection to attend my pain. To let goodness be a compassionate resource to the trauma I had experienced so long ago.

This, all of this, is the work of becoming strong like water.

{}

EMBODIED EXPERIENCES OF COMPASSIONATE WITH-NESS

That day in my old house, I had an *embodied experience*: I was fully present to my suffering, *and* I also experienced connection to Brendan's profound support. When we feel safe enough in our bodies to actually be present in and to them, moment to moment, our systems are fully "online"[2] and we have the capacity to live in our God-given bodies, wholly and fully.

Maybe it seems like I'm splitting hairs here; after all, it seems obvious that humans are embodied (or, to put it another way, we always seem to be *in body*). But the truth is, being present in our bodies makes a pretty big difference. Think how often we go on autopilot or get "stuck in our head" as we examine an idea. Consider how many of us have been taught it's better to stick with the "facts" whenever a situation brings up emotion. We live in a culture that frequently objectifies, commodifies, and quantifies bodies. When we treat ourselves and others like we are static objects—machines relying solely on rational thought—rather than image bearers with actual *bodies* and emotions, we don't have capacity to truly connect with what's happening in and through us. We learn to disconnect from our bodies as a default way to be in the world.

This is a particular danger for trauma survivors. Because our bodies are the physical location where the trauma is held, we may find it *necessary* to remain disconnected from them simply so we can function from day to day. That makes total

{}

sense, and we can honor that part of us that has had to work so hard to survive.

At the same time, as we do the sacred work of healing and experience more and more moments of true embodiment—of security and hope—it begins to change us. As I packed up my childhood home with Brendan's help, it felt extremely familiar to me to be in pain; it felt normal to feel as if I would have to figure out everything on my own and to stuff my feelings. What *didn't* feel natural was to sense deep validation and companionship in the midst of my pain; to have someone *with* me.

Now, let me be clear: The gift of presence that Brendan gave me earlier in our marriage was not based on his ability to save me. Frankly, he can't and he couldn't. I love him dearly, but he is just a person with limits and wounds himself.

What he could offer, though, was what I've come to call "compassionate with-ness," a posture through which others convey that they are attuned to us—that they resonate with, understand, and share our feelings—and that we can attune to them and to others. Hopefully this makes it possible for us to begin to learn to attune to ourselves as well. In Latin, the word *compassion* means to "suffer with." Suffering *with* someone while being attuned to them is powerful; it conveys a sacred solidarity. This with-ness also speaks to the way our nervous systems and bodies are created to sync with each other as we experience co-regulation.

This is the key difference between the idea of a "witness" and "with-ness": A witness can observe what has happened—which certainly matters. But "with-ness" implies that the person has resolved to be in it with us, right down in the dirt and mire of whatever we're going through. This is what Brendan did for me as I sat and cried on my parents' old couch. He was *with* me. Not just physically, but emotionally. He himself was embodied as he tuned in to my suffering, and he cared about it. Critically, he was also grounded himself, which enabled him to be calm, curious, and kind with me. And his tiny offering became the fertile ground for me to learn to become strong in new and unfamiliar ways.

Those moments of deep safety and co-regulation began to shift my internal narratives, sensations, and experiences in ways I could never have believed.

THE STRENGTH IN EMBODIMENT

Having someone see and help you hold your pain can be a revelation for you, too, if you hold a story in your body that tells you something like the following:

- *Your pain doesn't matter.*
- *You're not allowed to feel.*
- *You're selfish to feel.*
- *You're too much if you feel.*
- *You're alone in your pain.*

Not only that, but from a neurobiological view, simply being in the presence of another person's grounded nervous system can help expand your own window of tolerance.[3] And when you have numerous experiences of emotional, physical, and spiritual safety, your body will begin to sense that it can change its posture toward itself, your pain, your people, and your God.

Experiencing Brendan's patient attunement to my emotional state was what therapist Deb Dana refers to as a "necessary disconfirming experience that interrupts habitual neuroceptive responses."[4] In other words, those moments were the opposite of what my system had learned to expect. A surprise. A pivot point to create a new path forward. The world wasn't perfect, but I could access strength by learning to co-regulate and draw resources from my safe connection with him.

I believe the Pharisee Saul's experience on the road to Damascus is another powerful illustration of the power of embodied experiences. At the time, Saul—better known now as the apostle Paul—hated Jesus and persecuted His followers. But then Saul had a wild encounter with the resurrected Jesus. As he embarked on another mission to round up Christians, Jesus stopped him with a blinding light and said, "Saul, Saul, why do you persecute me?" (Acts 9:4).

After that experience, Saul *got it*. He'd had an embodied experience of the risen Jesus, and he couldn't help but talk about it and change his life accordingly. It certainly mattered that Saul was embodied, but what he experienced *while* embodied was also important. It was the combination of Saul being present to the radical disruption and experiencing the goodness and fullness of Jesus that created the true shift.

It's from this place that we begin to form a different template for how to understand God, others, and ourselves.

ATTACHMENT STYLES

DISMISSIVE

(Avoidant Attachment)

- *Tend to be self-reliant*
- *Are most afraid of feeling "engulfed" by other people*
- *Tend to be critical of others but less critical of themselves*
- *Are emotionally disconnected*
- *Are typically triggered by conflict; react by isolating to try to emotionally self-regulate*
- *Experience the most activation from their dorsal vagal complex when triggered by relationships*

PREOCCUPIED

(Anxious-Ambivalent Attachment)

- *Tend to desire validation and closeness*
- *Are most afraid of abandonment*
- *Are hypercritical of self but more apt to see others as "good"*
- *Tend to be emotionally dysregulated when fearing relational disconnection*
- *Are typically triggered by conflict and react by wanting more closeness*
- *Experience the most engagement from their sympathetic nervous systems (fight/flight/fawn) when triggered[5]*

FEARFUL-AVOIDANT

(Disorganized Attachment)

- *Desire to connect to other people but also fear being used and hurt*
- *Are most afraid that those closest to them will cause them harm*
- *Tend to see themselves as defective and others as scary*
- *May feel they are inviting others in while also pushing them out*
- *Tend to be emotionally dysregulated, which may result in dissociation and/or sympathetic nervous system activation*
- *Current relationships may activate a sense of terror rooted in previous disturbing relational experiences.*

AUTONOMOUS

(Secure Attachment)

- *Tend to be interdependent and able to connect with others and themselves*
- *Can acknowledge their own faults while also hearing their partners' concerns*
- *Are better able to stay emotionally regulated in everyday situations involving relationships*
- *Are able to more accurately assess whether a person is safe or reliable based on their previous experiences*

Strong like Water Language for Honoring Each Other's Needs

If it feels like a resource, I invite you to brainstorm together (with a romantic partner, family member, or friend) on what it might look like to honor the needs of both of you based on your own attachment style. It might sound like this:

If you have an avoidant style

"Sometimes when we have conflict or there is a lot of emotion, I find myself disconnecting or even getting angry. I'm working on listening to my body and knowing how to process emotions, but I'd like to know how you feel when you sense me responding that way.

Can we come up with a middle way to honor your needs while still enabling me to take breaks when I'm too overwhelmed?"

If you have an anxious style

"Sometimes when I don't hear back from you immediately, I start to panic, even though I know you care about me. What is it like for you when you sense me responding that way?

STRONG LIKE WATER THROUGH ATTACHMENT

In *Try Softer*, we spend a lot of time exploring how we each hold attachment styles based on early relationships with our primary caregivers.[6] Of course, these attachment styles can certainly shift based on other primary relationships we experience, and they are, in fact, fluid templates that change based on experiences and even the state of our nervous system. That being said, we each likely have a primary attachment style (see page 93), that can inform us about our relationship with God, others, and ourselves.

Once we know our primary attachment style, we can begin to imagine what kind of compassionate resources might move us along the flow of strength toward integration. Each style has different strategies for responding in situational strength—and therefore can be empowered to choose different strategies and rhythms in their journey to become strong like water.[7] As you'll see, for these healing strategies (which are not exhaustive and may overlap), I've indicated where in the book you can go to learn more if you wish. Additionally, if you are drawn to strategies from multiple attachment styles, I encourage you to experiment with whatever feels like a resource to you.

Avoidant attachment

This attachment style is typically indicative of those whose caregiver(s) or primary adult relationships are emotionally distant or cold. Often the caregiver will meet their children's physical needs but allow emotional needs to go unmet. And as a result, these kiddos learn that they must deal with difficult experiences or emotions on their own.

Fear: Overwhelm/engulfment by the emotions of another
- *It's not safe to feel.*
- *I have to do it alone.*

Situational strength strategy: Suppress/use anger to shut down/isolate/think instead of feel. May have difficulty remaining emotionally regulated when faced with big feelings because they did not receive support and care.

Can we come up with a middle way to honor your needs while still enabling me to build trust whenever we have distance?"

If you have a disorganized style

"Even though I know we care about each other, sometimes when I connect with you, it activates feelings of past trauma. It helps a lot to have you affirm that it's good for me to take care of myself and set boundaries in the way that I need. But what is it like for you when you sense me responding that way?

Can we come up with a middle way to honor your needs while still enabling me to build safety?"

Strong-like-water strategies
- Build awareness of WOT and notice when feelings or situations seem too overwhelming (chapter 2)
- Track body states (chapter 3)
- Understand what feels safe to your body (chapter 3)
- Titrate/ease into feelings (chapter 7)
- Listen to, speak on behalf of, and provide reparative experiences for your younger self (chapters 5 and 6)

Anxious attachment

This attachment strategy is developed when a caregiver(s) or a person's primary adult relationships are attuned inconsistently. Sometimes there is attunement, but the rest of the time the caregiver is deeply unavailable, dysregulated, or misattuning. When this happens, children learn that love is not consistent or reliable.

Fear: Abandonment
- *It's not safe to be alone.*
- *Everyone is going to leave—I need to keep them here as long as I can.*

Situational strength strategy: May use big emotion, fawning, or self-abandonment to stay connected to their attachment figure (parent, partner, friend), even at the cost of their authenticity or safety.

Strong-like-water strategies
- Build awareness of WOT and notice when feelings or situations seem to trigger a fear of abandonment (chapter 2)
- Soothe younger self when overwhelmed
  - grounding (chapter 1)
  - relational with-ness (chapter 4)
  - ART: Attune/Respond/Tend (chapter 5)
- Understand what feels safe to your body (chapter 3)
- Listen to, speak on behalf of, and provide reparative experiences for your younger self (chapters 5 and 6)
- Notice if or when you are drawn to "leaving yourself" in order to maintain connection with another person
- Explore adding some small distance to a relationship, and observe what it's like to safely return (e.g., don't immediately respond to a text and notice that it doesn't harm the relationship)
- Titrate/ease into feelings (chapter 7)

Disorganized attachment[8]

When children experience their caregivers as terrifying or as the source of their trauma, or when adults experience those closest to them as the source of a major disturbance, they are in a double bind—they want to experience connection but also fear it.

Fear: Connection is terrifying, but so is the sense of abandonment

- *Nothing feels safe.*
- *I want to be closer, but I am frightened by that possibility.*

Situational strength strategy: Remain isolated and alone and/or deeply dysregulated around others, despite desire for connection. May experience higher rates of dissociation (numbing/ zoning out) as well as all manner of trauma responses because the body does not know whether to move toward or away from connection.

This attachment style is especially prone to going into a freeze response. This often feels like having one foot on the gas and the other on the brake at the same time. As a result, pacing is critical; steps toward attachment should be small to provide the best combination of safety and growth.

Strong-like-water strategies

- Build a sense of safety through containment and grounding (chapter 1)
- Grow awareness of WOT—notice when feelings or situations seem too overwhelming or trigger fear of abandonment, harm, and/or a mixture of any of those emotions (chapter 2)
- Understand what feels safe to your body (chapter 3)
- Gently explore moving through emotions (chapter 7)

- Practice pendulation, which is tolerating small amounts of comfort and then pairing the comfort with small amounts of difficulty (chapter 7)
- Listen to, speak on behalf of, and provide reparative experiences for your younger self (chapters 5 and 6)

Secure attachment

When children experience "good enough" caregiving, their body's template reflects a realistic and secure view of the world. Generally speaking, people who experience a secure attachment have an innate sense that even when a rupture occurs, they will find a way to work it out.[9]

As I've said, our attachment styles are fluid templates that can change. This means that a person could begin life with an insecure attachment and have it shift to a secure one.[10] The opposite can also occur: A person has a secure attachment in early life, but after experiencing intense insecure attachment with a spouse or in another key relationship, their attachment could shift to insecure. In general, folks with a secure attachment are better positioned to intuitively tap into strong-like-water strategies, and yet each of us are human and can experience difficulty doing so.

Fear: Connection is to be expected, but it's not always easy to repair.

Situational strength strategy
- *It's difficult to be a human, and sometimes I act in ways that don't line up with who I truly am.*

Strong-like-water strategies
- Notice what's already working in your relationships
  - Resourcing (chapter 6)
- Look for opportunities to co-regulate with a romantic partner, friends, and/or family
- Practice emotional regulation and compassionately resource as you move along the spectrum of strength
- Practice repairing ruptures in relationships
- Recognize that others you care about may have a different attachment style
- Practice asking for what you need and communicating with others about their needs

THE WITH-NESS OF GOD

It's almost evening and the winter sun is setting. Light pinks and cool blues are strewn across the sky as I set off on a walk. I'm more tired and worn-out than I've been for a long time, as so many people are several months into the pandemic. Brendan knows I often need a bit of time to be by myself and move after being with my kiddos all day while (bless my heart) I attempt to homeschool. I'm finding it harder than I anticipated, even while being grateful it was an option for us after schools shut down. On top of that, I'm doing what

I can to manage my private therapy practice and my work as an author. It's a lot.

I'm processing so much and recognizing in a new way the cost of my childhood. I realize how normal it can feel for me to be isolated from others. I've done a lot of work to believe I am worth taking care of, but the reality remains: I've spent a lot of my life with people while still feeling profoundly alone. This, on top of the amount of suffering in the world right now, makes everything feel overwhelming and enormous.

But beauty hunting often brings me back to myself. So I pause at the corner for a moment to take in the views of the Rocky Mountains. I am captivated by what I see; as I settle into observing the snowcapped peaks, my shoulders lower and my breath settles. My heart, mind, body, and soul feel aligned—even if only for that moment.

My feet hit the pavement again, and my lips move in silent prayers: *God, give me eyes to see the ways You're already here. God, You're with me. You're with us.* I pray and sense God's nearness. And as I do, I feel a strength I can't fully explain. I'm not happy about any of the pain or hardship, and I know God doesn't celebrate my pain or anyone else's either. But I see something in a way I never have before: The with-ness of God and the with-ness of others are what create the framework for what makes us truly strong.

In some ways, I already know this. I've spoken and written about ideas like healing, wholeness, resilience, and compassion for a long time. Yet for some reason on this walk, it feels like a blurry telescope coming into new focus.

I think about Psalm 23, a favorite of mine:

The LORD is my shepherd, I lack nothing.
    He makes me lie down in green pastures,
he leads me beside quiet waters,
    he refreshes my soul.
He guides me along the right paths
    for his name's sake.
Even though I walk
    through the darkest valley,
I will fear no evil,
    for you are with me;
your rod and your staff,
    they comfort me.

You prepare a table before me
    in the presence of my enemies.
You anoint my head with oil;
    my cup overflows.
Surely your goodness and love will follow me
    all the days of my life,
and I will dwell in the house of the LORD
    forever.

The Hebrew word for the phrase "he leads me" in verse 2 is *nahal*, a verb that according to *Strong's Concordance* means "to lead or guide to a watering place, bring to a place of rest, refresh."[11] The Hebrew word for "quiet," *menuchah*, is a noun that means "resting place" or "rest."[12] So we have a God who tends us and leads us to the places that allow us to experience rest and refreshment.

Indeed, the Hebrew term translated "my shepherd" is a form of the word *ra'ah*, which means "to tend."[13] This is a God of connection; a God of co-regulation. A God who builds safety *in us and through us* because this connection is available to us. Because He is *with* us. Note that the shadows don't disappear and the enemies are still present at the table. Yet God's witness sustains the psalmist.

And I pray you experience the reality that He sustains you too.

Reader, you've been taught to view fear as a character flaw, but it's not. Fear is appropriate in situations that are unsafe or overwhelming. The invitation here is not to pretend that there is nothing to fear (because that doesn't actually work anyway). Instead, we are invited to sink into the presence of One who can help us navigate the fear. God joins us. Emmanuel joins us. God *with* us is the clearest invitation to secure attachment we could ever hope for.

What I realized anew looking at the splendor of the Rocky Mountains that day is that *connection is the remedy.* Connection with myself. Connection with others. Connection with God. Connection is what creates enough safety for you and me to move along the flow of strength. It's this flexibility, not the rigidity of stress or trauma, that makes us strong. Connection is what expands into hope, courage, and life. Psychiatrist Gabor Maté speaks to the interplay between safety and connection when he says, "Safety is not the absence of threat, but the presence of connection."[14]

This is why it matters in such a profound way that God, in the person of Jesus, came to be near us; came to take on humanity and defeat death. God *came* for us and to be *with us*: Jesus, Emmanuel, God with us. This is the power of the Incarnation. It's not that God didn't love us before Christ came, but in the same way my loving attunement to my children communicates something important, so too does God's physical presence here on earth.

God knows we are fragile. He knows how our bodies function and move into stress responses and pain. As someone who has experienced chronic attachment trauma, I can confidently say I notice when someone turns toward me. When they come for me. When they honor and care for me, while still honoring my voice and personhood. And I believe this is what God did, what God is like.

By taking on flesh, Jesus didn't give us merely a spiritual answer to the complexity of our humanity. He didn't spiritually bypass His humanity either. Instead, God took on flesh and said, in effect, *This is how far I'll go to love you.*

So of course—of course—the truest, deepest strength would follow this same model. The strength to move through pain, harm, and trauma is found in connection and ultimately safety; with God, ourselves, others, and creation. When we really know this, it allows us to move along the spectrum from situational strength toward transitional strength and ultimately toward a deep integrated strength. When we feel connected, we have the support to be more fully ourselves.

Honestly, if that's not grace—I don't know what is.

BECOMING STRONG LIKE WATER
DEVELOPING RELATIONAL WITH-NESS

Take a moment to consider someone in your life whom you have experienced as reliable, calming, supportive, or kind (they could be all of these). If you can't think of anyone whom you've experienced in this way, that's okay. In fact, this is normal for many trauma survivors. If you have experienced God in this supportive way, you may also choose to invite Him into the exercise.

(One caveat: Though you may have faith in God, I invite you to assess whether it feels helpful to invite Him into this space, depending on your level of felt safety with Him. You'll recall that earlier I shared that though I've had a strong faith in God my entire life, it wasn't until I'd experienced safety with people that I could begin to transfer that template to God. If this is true for you, too, I encourage you to remember that God's goodness presents itself in so many ways, including through the people who love and care about us.)

If you need additional connections that feel safe, consider a character from a show or book who may have these traits. You might bring to mind an animal, pet, or even an object that has felt comforting to you (e.g., a blanket, candle, or book).

Once you've chosen a connection, take a moment to ground yourself in the space you're in, which will bring you into your WOT and feeling neutral and/or resourced. Next, with either a soft gaze or eyes closed, consider one of the people you've thought of as a support. As you're able, bring them into your mind's eye.

What do you notice about them? Does it feel good, pleasant, supportive, or calming to have them with you? Or do you notice your nervous system becoming activated in a way that does not feel supportive? If so, I invite you to pause and try this practice again with a different support.

If you find that the support you are connecting with feels like a resource (e.g., your body continues to feel grounded and/or calm, present, focused, relaxed, known, etc.), I invite you to continue this practice.

Now, notice:

- Where is your supportive ally in proximity to you as you visualize them: next to you, behind you, beside you, far away from you?[15] If you like where they are, wonderful. If you would like them to be in a different proximity to you, prompt them to move so that their presence feels more supportive.

- Do they say anything to you? Does this feel helpful? If not, remember you can change how this unfolds.

- Do they do anything? Is this supportive? If not, remember you can have them change how they act to better help you.

PSALM 23: HE LEADS US BESIDE STILL WATERS

Psalm 23 has long been a resource to me. I see its imagery as an invitation to experience security with God as we are able. However, if for any reason reflecting on this Scripture does not feel supportive to your body and system, I invite you either to let it go or to shift this exercise in ways that feel helpful. Additionally, if at any point this becomes overwhelming or flooding to your system, please discontinue and use other resources such as grounding, containment, or orienting.

1. To begin, I invite you to ensure you feel grounded and connected to your WOT. Now take a moment to reread Psalm 23. (You may consider looking at alternate Bible versions.)

2. Notice any verses that stand out to you. As you consider this, I invite you to be aware of what is coming up in your body. What is the quality of your breath? Where do you notice sensations in your body? What emotions do you feel?

3. If it feels helpful, place a hand or hands on your heart or any area that you sense would benefit from that embodied support. As you do this, what emotions do you feel?

4. Does this practice continue to feel like a resource? If so, take a moment, and place yourself in the imagery from the psalm that feels supportive. How is God attending to you? Does it feel possible to receive this care? If so, I invite you to savor that sensation. If not, could you place someone you deeply care about in the scene with you? Can they receive the care? If so, would it be possible to allow yourself to sit alongside this person and receive the care with them?

5. I invite you to stay with this resource as long as it feels helpful to you. Remember that you can always return to this practice.

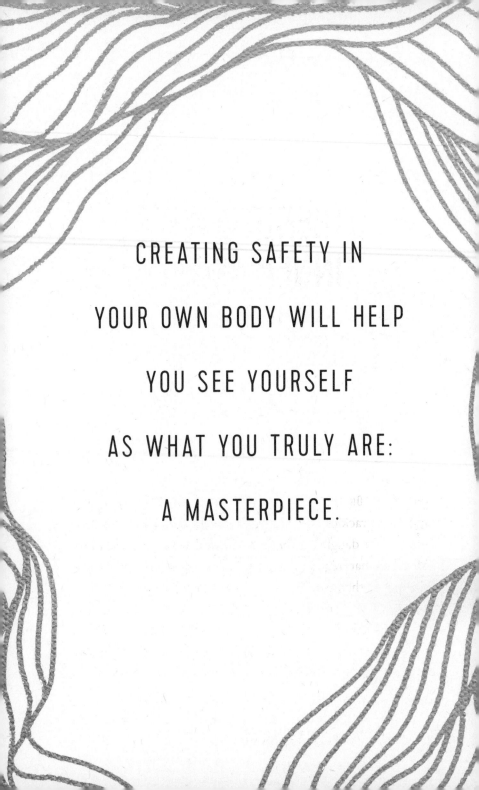

CREATING SAFETY IN

YOUR OWN BODY WILL HELP

YOU SEE YOURSELF

AS WHAT YOU TRULY ARE:

A MASTERPIECE.

CHAPTER 5

STRENGTH WITH INNER TRUST

For some of us, warrior mode is easy.
Tenderness is hard. Healing shifts the heart.

DR. THEMA BRYANT

I'M SITTING ON THE FLOOR OF OUR SHOWER, sobbing. The baby monitor crackles and hums in the background. Our six-month-old daughter, Tia, is lovely and wondrous with big blue eyes that frequently stop me in my tracks—but I haven't slept more than two hours straight since her birth. My mom came to town for several weeks after her birth, and I bawled when she left. Though we've had a complicated relationship for many years, I am seeing in a new way how she continues to show up and repair our relationship in the ways she can.

That doesn't change how frayed and ragged I am right now, however. Both "tired and wired," as the saying goes. My anxiety makes me feel like someone plugged me into a damaged electrical socket. My well-worn armor of achievement, hustling, and appeasing others is useless here, as I'm adjusting to motherhood.

But. Every day when my little one takes her exactly-thirty-eight-minute nap, I come and sit in the shower, letting the warmth and comfort envelop my body. A brief moment of goodness.

The tears let up, and I catch my breath. In most respects, I don't know why I'm crying anymore. Cognitively, I know that it's partly my body readjusting after the birth of my baby. But it also feels deeper, like parts of my story—the unhealed wounds of my own childhood—are calling me to listen. Asking me to pay attention. I am not quite sure how to do that yet. All I know for sure is that giving myself a chance to be nourished—even in this small way of letting myself cry in the shower—feels right.

As time goes on, I slowly, ever so slowly, begin to find my way as a mother. I make a few mom friends; Brendan and I start to develop a rhythm as a family of three; I get back into therapy to confront the postpartum anxiety and depression that have set in. And in therapy, I begin to unpack a layer of my story I didn't know was there: the extent to which I had simply survived much of my life rather than lived it before Tia was born. I understand, on a deeper level, the high cost of all the times I had to be situationally strong.

It takes a lot of work, but at the same time that I learn how to be a mother to my daughter, I learn what it means to mother myself—to father myself too. Not because I don't need anyone else; of course I do. But for the first time in my life, instead of feeling as if all the safety available to me comes from *outside* my body—my husband, God, a few safe friends—I begin to see that somewhere *in me* is a soft landing place as well. It is like the love and safety I have experienced with Brendan, with my Jesus, and with a few safe people begin to form in me a new center—one of embodied, internalized safety.

Here, in what feels like a tumultuous storm brought on by new motherhood, I find a new inner trust, which leads to a new inner strength. All the aching parts of myself are beginning to speak up, to let me know the extent of the pain they have carried for so long—and instead of ignoring them, acting like the pain isn't real, I get quiet. I don't try to hustle my way out of discomfort or shame myself for feeling disconnected. Though it feels fragile and new, I finally start to listen.

And there I find that my truest, wisest, most compassionate self is finally ready to speak up too. And boy, is she fierce.

RESOURCING OUR WAY TO INNER STRENGTH

Throughout the book, we've emphasized the value and necessity of safety. And yet this idea of *internalized* safety is an important step in our strong-like-water work because it's often an indication that we are beginning to operate out of *transitional strength*, that liminal space between situational and integrated strength in the flow. Witnessing the blossoming of this skill is one of the best parts of my job as a therapist: It's a profound honor to watch a client begin to have a sense—even a glimpse—of this soft landing place within themselves.

How do we begin to trust ourselves like this? Initially it may feel vulnerable to engage the work of listening to our inner lives, especially if we didn't receive the care we needed from our parents or caregivers. And certainly, as we've already discussed, developing this internal soft landing place doesn't mean we can do the work of life on our own, or that we don't need the God who helps us hold it all—but it does mean that we are invited to *participate* in our own lives. Throughout the Bible we see evidence that our God compassionately cares and attends to us; and in so doing, God empowers us to steward this care toward ourselves too.

So when we experience these new emotional shifts on the inside, how do we use them to influence our world on the outside? There are several ways for us to integrate internalized safety, but one of the most salient channels I know is through resourcing, or compassionately connecting to internal or external forms of support to meet whatever challenges we face. Instead of forcing ourselves to be situationally strong, to push through, no matter the cost, we realize that resources are lifelines—salient moments we return to, relational connections, or skills we pick up along the way that we can lean on when life begins to feel like too much. These resources could be as simple as doing a grounding exercise when you're feeling off, saying a breath prayer, or having a plan of who to call when your day has tanked. They could be as complex as creating scripts to navigate difficult boundary conversations or getting outside to move so you can fully process your emotions. What's important in each of these examples is how the resource is experienced by *your body*. What is a support for one person may not be for another—and that's okay. This is why so much of this work is not about following a checklist but having internal conversations. It bears repeating that having resources doesn't and can't replace support that is meant to be met by a community—but ultimately we need support both externally *and* internally.

Having a set of resources in my toolbox allowed me to tune in to my needs in those early days of motherhood. It wasn't because I could do it all on my own (I couldn't!) but because without acknowledging and engaging my inner landscape, I was woefully ill-equipped to ask for what I needed, let alone act on it. So whenever I noticed myself becoming overwhelmed or activated, choosing a resource would often be the pivot point I needed to both honor where I was *and* find strength to move through it.

This was also true for my client Jenna, who grew up gaining lots of external praise academically and even socially from just about everyone—except the one person she ached to hear it from: her mom. If Jenna got an A on a

Signs You Might Be Experiencing Transitional Strength

· Growing sense of internalized safety (an internal soft landing place)
· Awareness that two things can be true at once (both/and)
· Acceptance of more nuance. *Hello, gray area!*
· Increasing sense of a full spectrum of emotions. *So you're saying there are more than two emotions?*
· Ability to observe your own experience (to "think about thinking"[1])
· Greater awareness of your own limits. *Yeah, that's not going to work for me.*
· Increasing ability to connect with your body. *I'm noticing a sensation in my . . .*
· A sense of common humanity;[2] awareness of not being alone. ("You are not the only one who feels like the only one.")[3]
· Increasing ability to mindfully connect with resources. *Remember the other time I got through that hard thing?*

paper, her mother scathingly asked why it wasn't an A+. If Jenna's hair was out of place, she called her daughter horrid names. Whenever Jenna became excited about a cause or an idea, she knew she would have to bury her passion so that her mom wouldn't find a way to take it from her. As a result of her mom's verbal abuse, Jenna struggled with a deeply held belief that she was worthless; a failure. In fact, for many years Jenna thought her inner critic was normal and if she wasn't such a failure, her inner critic wouldn't make her want to crawl in a hole and disappear. This critic could be brutal, making Jenna shut down and disengage from her present life completely—in much the same way she had as a teenager.

We had worked together for about a year before she sat down on the couch in my office one day and told me, "Aundi, the weirdest thing happened this last week. While I was riding my bike downtown, I got distracted and crashed into another biker. And it was absolutely my fault. I should have been more careful.

114

Luckily, we were both wearing helmets and were totally okay.

"But here's where it started to get interesting: In a situation like this, I would usually be a total disaster, diving headlong into a massive shame spiral at my mistake. And, of course, it was so stressful that I started to notice my body getting incredibly anxious. But *this time*, instead of hearing the voice of my raging inner critic, which sounds an awful lot like my mom, I heard . . . well, yours."

A smile crossed my lips, because I absolutely knew what she meant. Other clients have told me this before, and in my own life, I've heard the voices of others in similar moments.

Jenna started to smile too. "I mean, it wasn't, like, in a creepy way. But as I felt the anxiety begin to rise, I remembered how you often say to me in a session, 'And what is your body saying you might need right now?' And in that moment, I was able to take a deep breath and just settle myself. Yes, I made a mistake, but no one was hurt. And I was capable of finding a solution, despite the stress.

- Expanding ability to down-regulate and up-regulate the nervous system. *When I'm anxious I could try X; when I feel depressed, I could try Y.*
- Increasing ability to self-soothe. *It's okay to take care of myself when I'm in pain.*
- Initial move toward interdependence. *I am capable of listening to my needs and it's okay to need others.*
- Connection as an increasingly common resource. *I don't have to do this alone.*

115

I knew—I just knew—that even though it was hard, I was capable of moving through this hard thing."

Wow, what a beautiful moment to witness. By honoring her reality *and* accessing a compassionate inner resource, Jenna was laying the foundation of a new phase of her healing process: She was beginning to build internalized safety. When the crash occurred, she could have let her inner critic rehash the accident over and over so she wouldn't make a mistake like that again. In some ways, her body knew this pattern well; after all, one way her body had adapted so it could stay one step ahead of her mom and survive her childhood was by developing this inner critic. But because of the work Jenna had done with me in therapy, she was beginning to understand that, if left untended, this crash could get stuck in her body as trauma, and the cycle of unhealed pain might continue.

Indeed, Jenna was at a crossroads: She could let her critic lead the way—or she could choose a new path. She could choose to pay compassionate attention to her needs, even in stress. She could choose herself.

"When I got home, I still felt really shaky," Jenna continued. "So I practiced being kind to myself. First, I did a grounding exercise just like we've practiced, and then I took a hot shower while I listened to a few songs that always make me feel like myself.

"After that, I called my neighbor Daniella and asked if she wanted to watch a movie with me; I just needed to be near another person, you know? It wasn't perfect, by any means.

But I did it," Jenna finished. Her eyes were bright with tears and hope.

Reader, this is my desire for you too.

Learning to experience, steward, and ultimately leverage the safety we experience through connection with God, self, and others is where the mystery and goodness of strong like water is truly born.

REPARENTING: GETTING IT RIGHT

We each have our own unique experiences from childhood—both wounds and treasures. As we discussed in chapter 4, our attachment styles give us information about our templates when it comes to relationships, ourselves, and even God. Ideally, we've experienced "good enough" parenting, which helps us form a template of internalized safety that can help us regulate, self-soothe, and experience satisfying connection. Yet experts estimate nearly 50 percent of people have insecure attachment styles and so feel disconnected from this internal support.[4]

As we engage the work of becoming strong like water, we can learn to attune to the ways our bodies have done their best to help us adapt to a lack of support. We can learn to honor, soothe, and listen to the pain that presents itself as we lovingly assess what we need and participate with God to give it to ourselves. This is *reparenting*—and it's a great resource to draw upon as we engage the work of healing.

Building internalized safety with ourselves looks like

honoring where we came from—honoring why we attach the way we do—and then doing what we can to meet ourselves where we are. And though this is internal work, we are not alone. We are held and loved by the God of the universe. As the psalmist aptly wrote, "Your love, LORD, reaches to the heavens, your faithfulness to the skies" (Psalm 36:5).

Indeed.

With that said, let's build on what we've already learned about our attachment styles to see how the resource of internalized safety can expand our capacity and move us along the flow of strength. Before we begin, we need to remember that attachment styles are fluid and, even more importantly, that they are not a diagnosis. They're simply the strategies we use to get our needs met. Yet if we can see them as the invitations they are to explore our stories, we can learn to lean in with compassion for the wounds we hold.

A few more suggestions: As you consider and work with each attachment style, you may wish to notice how old you feel when you think about it.[5] For example, if thinking about needing to isolate makes you feel as though you are around five years old, you might imagine yourself at that age. As you do, consider asking this younger part of yourself if any of the statements below feel helpful or nurturing. If for any reason your younger self is not ready to connect with your present self, or if the situational strength you've used to survive is not yet open to being influenced by your adult self's presence, that's okay. We always want to honor the pace of our bodies, remembering that as trust is built, the internal relationship will strengthen and over time will be open to more connection.

Avoidant attachment

If you identify strongly with having an avoidant attachment style, you may feel like all your physical needs were adequately taken care of—but that emotional care was never part of the gig. Because that is true, you likely experienced a lack of emotional support, warmth, and attunement from your caregivers.

If this happened, your brilliant body naturally adapted, and this may have resulted in an overdeveloped left hemisphere of your brain (which values logic, analytics, and facts) and/or a lesser developed right brain (which helps us connect with nuance, intuition, creativity, our emotions, and our bodies).[6] This may be why any display of emotions—whether your own or other people's—and any sense of conflict in relationship may instantaneously feel overwhelming, though outwardly it may appear as though you don't care or that you are even irritated or angry.

As a child, you may have come to believe that emotional needs were a liability that led to shame, isolation, and neglect. You may have learned that the valid emotional support you needed to help you navigate the world just wasn't there. So now when a relationship becomes emotionally charged, you may feel a need to detach and isolate as a way to navigate the situation. If an emotion rises within you, you may consciously or unconsciously work to detach from that part of yourself, whether it's through numbing or avoidance. Basically, you'll do anything not to feel—feeling, you've learned, is a burden. Instead, you cope with the world by relying heavily on logic and thinking, believing you are the only person you can depend on anyway.

My dear reader, this makes sense. As you work to become strong like water, it will be important for you to honor this hurting part's pace and all the various situational strengths that have offered a sort of protection from pain.

Little by little, you'll begin to build a foundation of internalized safety. You will "witness and attune" to the younger part of yourself (located in your lower brain/amygdala) that wasn't nurtured emotionally.

With that in mind, consider these supportive statements for this particular style. If it would be a helpful resource, you might invite your adult self to speak these words over your younger self:

*I know it's felt safer to be alone. I want you to know that
 when you're ready, I'm here and I'm listening.*
*I know you've done it alone for a long time. Would it be okay
 if I tried to help?*
You can take your time with feeling; it's okay to pace yourself.
It is not weak to feel.
How can I support you?
Would it be okay if we let others support us too?
*It's okay to need space, and there's a lot of good from
 connection too.*
Can I help you receive goodness?

A RESOURCE TO PRACTICE

As you are able, see if you can notice when someone is truly supportive and follows through and does what they say they will. When this happens, you may be tempted to discount it and use a "deactivating" strategy such as ignoring or numbing the goodness that is actually present.[7] Though it may feel uncomfortable, see if you can let yourself recognize that it's okay to receive this kind of support.

When you notice this, observe how your body reacts to someone else's care. If it feels like a resource, in your mind's eye show your younger self this example of the ways you're not alone.

Anxious ambivalent attachment

If you learned to navigate relationships by consciously or unconsciously anticipating all the potential ways you could be abandoned, you likely have an anxious ambivalent attachment style.

Whereas a person with an avoidant style may experience anxiety about what therapist Diane Heller calls "approach stress," you may experience "departure stress," a sense of protest and grief over a connection seeming to end.[8] This stress is typically spurred by the implicit memories your body carries about all the ways connection with your caregiver(s) ultimately led to misattunement and aloneness.[9] As a child, you may have learned that attunement and care are not dependable—at best, they are intermittent and often followed by experiences of abandonment.

Because of this, any signs of conflict, space, or avoidance may feel terrifying to you. They may activate an anxiety rooted in the need to maintain connection *no matter what*. Importantly, this may be true even if you experienced many supportive and attuned interactions with your parents or caregivers. The key is that if they weren't *consistently* reliable, your body will still remember and organize itself around this reality.

Internally, and potentially unconsciously, you may also notice a desire for someone else to rescue you from your feelings, an experience, or even your life. Diane Heller notes that folks with an anxious ambivalent style tend to "rely . . . heavily on others to regulate their feelings."[10] This actually makes a lot of sense. Part of the goal of childhood is first to learn to co-regulate with a caregiver, which then helps us learn to self-regulate. However, with an anxious attachment style, the co-regulation was never fully accomplished because it was usually paired with abandonment—thus, this may have left you less equipped to self-regulate as an adult.

And yet, as we compassionately turn to these elements of our stories, we are equipped to remember that we can both need other people *and* listen to the ache inside ourselves. These signals from our body are telling us that a younger part of us needs care. If we can learn to recognize that this desire for outside support is valid, we'll find it's also an invitation to see and honor this hurting part of ourselves.

In doing this we can begin the process of communicating embodied safety to ourselves, through supportive statements such as:

I know so many people have left, but I will stay. (Adult self
    to hurting part)
I'm listening; I'm sorry there were so many times when I didn't.
Your feelings matter to me.
Even when others need space, it doesn't mean you're alone.
I am right here; how can I help?
It makes sense that you feel abandoned. Of course you do.
Can I help you receive goodness?
Would it be okay if I show you how things are different now?

A RESOURCE TO PRACTICE

As you are able, aim to notice when someone acts in a caring
manner toward you. See if you can give yourself permission
to truly savor the way they checked in with you, asked how
you are, provided care for you, or truly listened.

Observe how your body reacts to this care. If it feels like
a resource, in your mind's eye show your younger self this
example of the way that people *do* care for you.

Disorganized attachment

Each of us has a valid biological need for connection. Yet, if
you experience the difficult double bind of wanting people
close while simultaneously feeling scared or terrified of how
they'll hurt you, you may identify with a disorganized attachment style. Through repeated harmful experiences with those
who should have been the most present to you, you may have
learned that not only were they unavailable or misattuned,
they were often dangerous. This can happen when our parents

or caregivers are abusive or harm us in any way. But it can also happen when parents or caregivers have their own unresolved trauma, which may cause them to fear their children, have sudden intense mood swings, or become extremely unpredictable.[11] Either way, you may find it triggering both to move toward and away from someone, dear one.

A disorganized attachment may feel quite confusing both for you and for those who wish to connect with and love you, which makes a lot of sense. At times you may give signals that communicate "come closer; leave me alone." This pictures how you may feel with others, and it's a glimpse of your own internal world. You may experience simultaneous patterns of needing to get away from someone while concurrently feeling activated to move toward them. From a neurobiological perspective, we can often tolerate this tension for only so long before dissociating or moving into the freeze response. Again, that makes so much sense in the context of a childhood where you may have felt trapped, terrified, and deeply disoriented.

I want to recognize what a weight it is to carry any type of insecure attachment style, but particularly the immense pain that can come with an orientation toward a disorganized one. As someone who has in the past identified as anxious ambivalent but also as "situationally disorganized,"[12] I want you to know that it's quite normal to feel grief about this. At the same time, I want to offer you this hope: Even now, the work you are doing to learn about your body and your responses is beginning to lay the foundation for safety.

Below are several statements that may be a resource to you as you reparent and honor the pain you have carried:

I'm right here; I'll stay as close as feels good to you.
It's okay to feel whatever you feel; I won't leave.
I am listening.
I'd love to help however I can; what do you need?
You can take as much time as you need.
It makes sense that you feel scared. It was scary.
We can take this at your pace.
I know it's scary to connect with others sometimes. How can I help?
Let's work together to create boundaries that feel good to you.

A RESOURCE TO PRACTICE

First, take a moment to settle and ground your body. Then, as you are able, ask your younger self[13] who might be carrying the pain of the disorganized attachment if there is anyone this part of you feels is supportive to have alongside you as you consider the reparenting statements above (see relational allies resource on pages 105–107 and 147 for some ideas). You may find it helpful to bring in an ally who feels protective, or you may need to visualize an ally who is more nurturing—you could also do both.

If the feedback from your younger self is that no one feels helpful, I invite you to ask your younger self if you can offer them something that *would* feel comforting. For example, in your mind's eye you may wish to give this younger you a cozy blanket, a stuffed animal, or a cup of warm milk or tea. You could also do any of those actions for yourself in the present as well, which will also communicate comfort to your younger self. Our goal here is to continue building safety and trust with our younger selves, so our *responsiveness* to the information our younger self shares is key.

THE MERCY OF REPAIR

Building an internal sense of safety and trust, as well as safe connection with others, is hard and sacred work. It's key to beginning to understand and process the stories and unhealed wounds that have made us who we are. Not only that, but I have come to think of it as a great honor to have the opportunity to listen and tend to the wounds and situational strength that my younger self has carried for so long. And though I want to validate wherever you are in your own process, I want to invite you to see yourself through this framework too. Instead of being a great burden (though it may feel that way at times), what a great mercy it is that it's possible for us to repair it. Reader, if I could sit across from you right now, I would say: "Look at you doing this hard, beautiful work. Look at you. I'm so proud of you."

Finally, I want you to know I believe with every ounce of my being that your hard, tender work will not be in vain. Paradoxically, building this self-trust through truly caring and creating safety in your own body will pave the way to help you live and see yourself as what you truly are: a master-piece. Living art. Strong like water.

BECOMING STRONG LIKE WATER: LIVING ART

Recently I read this quote from Gregory of Nyssa: "Beauty is one of God's names." This statement felt so accurate that I felt goose bumps travel up my arms as I considered it. Beauty *is* one of God's names. And when we see something that moves us, stirs us, or causes us to feel deeply, it calls out something—perhaps the *imago Dei,* or image of God—in each of us.

Sometimes it can be hard to believe, but as Psalm 139:14 says, we are "fearfully and wonderfully made." We are art designed by the Artist.

This is part of what was on my mind as I developed the ART tool below. My hope is that it will provide language and tools to help us continue to reparent ourselves.

TOOLS FOR BUILDING SELF-TRUST AND SAFETY FOR OURSELVES

Attune

When you are grounded, nonjudgmentally (or even compassionately) attending and validating the experiences of your body opens you up to the practice of attunement.[14] In this first step, you can begin to name your experience. You may choose to simply notice the sensations in your body, and/or if it feels pertinent, add a description of feeling to those sensations. Additionally, you may wish to note your felt sense of the experience; in other words, its general theme.

For example, when I walk into my home after being away on a trip, I may smell a hint of eucalyptus. I then notice a sense of lightness in my chest as I finally place my bag on the floor. In that moment, I feel an overall sense of relief for finishing my travel and getting a chance to rest. However, let's say when I arrive home and set my bag on the floor, I suddenly notice a knot forming in my stomach and sense anxiety building as I remember all the emails I need to return. Next I remember that I have to get up early tomorrow and it's nearly bedtime. At this point, I may notice my sense of dread and overwhelm at being home.

Attunement itself is a vital part of building self-trust, but it also allows us to know how to respond to our own needs. In the example above, attunement helps me to know what my next steps might be. If I feel dread rather than relief, this can help me understand how to better care for myself as I move forward. Attunement equips us because we are tapping into the reality of what actually is.

Respond

Responding to your own needs is a vital part of practicing ART. Attunement can tell you what's going on and is in itself a form of response, but this next step is about mobilizing your energy to act on your own behalf. With this in mind, consider how you might respond to the information you've received from attuning. What do you need to fully engage?

To stay with the example from above, if I feel dread when I first return home, I might first practice some self-compassion.[15] By taking a moment to place a hand on my heart and my stomach where I feel the knot of anxiety, I acknowledge that this truly does feel hard. Perhaps it's been a long day, and there is a lot weighing on me about the week ahead. Then I might take a moment to ground and orient myself in my space and even acknowledge the reality that my needs matter too. As I do, I recognize that in my childhood, prioritizing other people's needs above my own valid needs was the way I survived. Noting that my body is settling even more and the knot in my stomach is beginning to soften, I might take a moment to acknowledge that none of the emails I need to send are urgent. Instead, I grab some water. I eat a snack. I give myself permission to go at the pace I need tonight. Each of these elements is a way I am mobilizing my energy to respond to myself in love. Your own experiences may differ from mine, but my hope is that you can begin to find ways to respond to your own needs in love too.

Tend

Once you begin learning how to respond to your own needs, you can move into tending them. In this final phase of ART, you keep an eye out for your needs while making yourself available to others. After I've eaten a snack and made the decision to wait until morning to review my emails, I am in a better place to sit down with Brendan to debrief about our day.

To better illustrate this phase, I'll use one of my mom hacks as an example. If I want to chat with a friend while we both have our kids with us, I've learned that it's helpful to meet at a playground (or someplace similar). That way, if Jude or Tia need me, I am absolutely available and am also aware of what they're doing at all times. However, I can also converse with my friend. Just as I'm present with and aware of my kids' activity at the park while I'm talking with my friend, once you are attuned and responsive to your most pressing needs, your body will likely not need you in quite the same way. But if it does, you will be *available* to respond. Now that you're connected to yourself, you can step back a bit, even as your willingness to be available to yourself when needed is a way you can build self-trust.

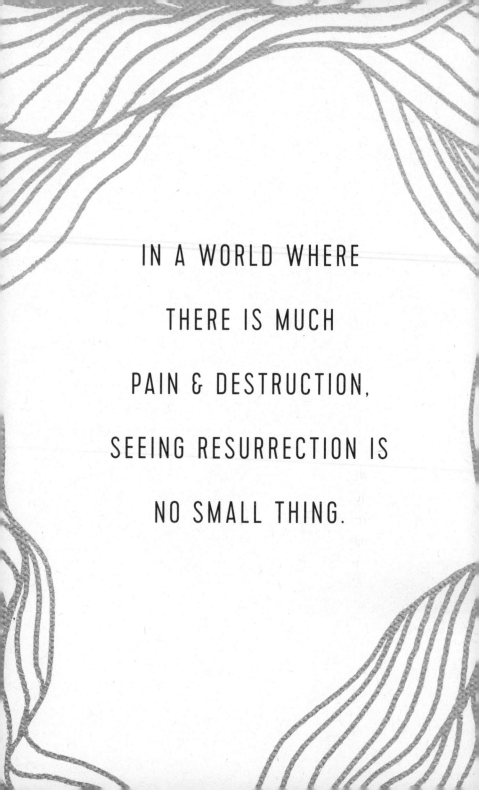

IN A WORLD WHERE

THERE IS MUCH

PAIN & DESTRUCTION,

SEEING RESURRECTION IS

NO SMALL THING.

CHAPTER 6

STRENGTH WITH GOODNESS

Even the gifts—especially the gifts—make sacred.

SARAH BLONDIN

"WOW, DO WE HAVE A LOT TO TALK ABOUT, AUNDI. A lot," Iris told me, slightly breathless as she plopped onto my couch at the start of our therapy session.

Like many of my clients, Iris had experienced chronic relational trauma throughout her childhood. Her father abused alcohol and her mother was rarely around. Iris's relational trauma was exacerbated when, in college, she experienced sexual violence in a setting where she should have felt safe—campus ministry. All of these experiences had affected Iris in multiple ways, including the shame she felt about her body; believing that somehow she was dirty and at fault for having been harmed. Our sessions over the past six months had focused on laying a foundation of safety by helping Iris become aware of her nervous system and begin internalizing a feeling of safety with herself. It had been hard and sacred work.

"Last week," Iris began, "I got a great promotion at work. My supervisor was so kind and spent a lot of time talking about how she experiences me in my role: how she sees me confidently presenting information, seeking out opportunities for growth, and taking the initiative to make those around me feel welcome. She finished her report by telling me, 'You're not hard to love, Iris.'"

I smiled; that was my experience with Iris too. She wasn't hard to love at all. "What a compliment," I agreed. "How did hearing that feel in your body?"

"It felt . . . a little odd. But also really good. I tried to connect with it a few other times during the week—the way we've practiced—and as I did, I began to remember how often I've felt hard to love. I have such compassion for that former me."

As Iris said this, I saw her sit up a little straighter. I noticed, too, that her shoulders were back; she had a steady look that I'd seen only a few times.

"Iris, as you're telling me this, what are you noticing?" I asked.

"Hmm," she replied, as she took a moment to consider my question. "The best way to describe it is that I feel like I can take up more space. I feel solid and . . . I notice a good weight in my chest."

What Iris was experiencing was the blooming of her transitional strength; her confidence was beginning to grow—and she was becoming aware of what that physically felt like in her body. As for many of us, Iris's work was not simple. It was layered and complex. But on this particular day, Iris's resources had an upward spiral effect, and she began to flow toward a new type of strength, her brain creating and strengthening new neural pathways. This enabled her to experience these pleasant emotions in ways she never had before. For maybe the first time in her life, Iris actually believed that she was not hard to love, and that meant *everything*.

SAVORING GOODNESS

A crucial part of healing from trauma—and ultimately in becoming who God created us to be—is being able to tap into resources of goodness. And yet it can be easy to assume that savoring what is good, right, and nourishing doesn't really matter. After all, why would it be important to take time to make sure we're truly experiencing the goodness in our lives? Isn't the point to heal and move forward, to fix the trauma and move on? *My life is stressful; I've got things to do; I've got decades of trauma to unlearn . . . and you want me to intentionally take time to stop and smell the flowers because that's* actually going to help?

The truth is, yes. Though it may feel counterintuitive, learning to connect to goodness is a part of what will actually allow us to heal. I don't say this carelessly. I know that for many of us, there is a lifetime of valid pain wrapped up in why we don't allow ourselves this grace; why goodness hasn't felt possible or accessible. But this reality remains: If we don't tenderly and compassionately tether ourselves to goodness, we remain disconnected from our truest healing.

And if we have lived the bulk of our lives in situational strength, one healing experience of safety isn't enough. A Band-Aid on a cannonball-sized wound won't do the trick. The repair has to match the wound. When we are speaking of the wounds trauma imprints on our bodies, experiences of safety are a vital piece of the repair. The more safety that is anchored in our bodies and the more positive experiences we have to draw from, the more intuitive it will become to stay within our windows of tolerance.

And so we must learn to resource. We must learn to fight to see—and hold tight to—goodness.

We've talked a lot about resourcing already, but it bears repeating: This is not an indulgence. This is not a "nice thing to do if I can get to it," a "Sure, I'll stop and appreciate the flowers if I have the time." This *is* the work, dear ones. And yes, we must honor the pace of our body, even as it's connected to goodness. But as I said to a client just the other day, "Resourcing isn't dessert; it's the meal." If you've experienced a lack of nurturing, soothing, and attuned relationships in your life—especially after traumatic experiences—it's as though your body has learned to operate on a vitamin deficiency. So to heal, we need to make sure your body has what it needs for the hard work ahead.

Imagine that you've signed up to run a marathon. Before now, running has not been a life priority—sure, you've got a pair of sneakers, you've logged a couple of two-mile jogs when the weather cooperates, but it hasn't been a consistent rhythm. If you just showed up to race day with that level of training . . . well, it's safe to say the next twenty-six miles wouldn't treat you well. It wouldn't be pretty—and it could even be really harmful to your body.

Instead, to run a marathon we have to train. We need the right "shoes" for our body. We need to know how to breathe, how to pace ourselves. We need to bank mile after mile after mile of practice. We need to prepare ourselves for what's ahead.

Resourcing is nourishing ourselves; it's *equipping*, but in the most paradoxical way: not with pain, but with goodness. In the marathon of life, if our brains and nervous systems are compassionately resourced, we become more resilient as we process pain.

It's as though the resources create Bubble Wrap around all the fragile pieces of us and help hold us together. This is a great picture of what resourcing in general does for us. It's not wasteful or a denial of reality to intentionally cultivate glimmers of goodness and experiences of safety in our body. Instead, those glimmers of life *are* what will help us find a way through.

OFF TO THE LAKE

Though my husband grew up in the Chicagoland area, the lakes of western Michigan created the backdrop of much of his childhood. Kolber family legend says that over fifty years ago when my father-in-law was in high school, he helped his father build a humble lake cottage. And from that, a whole family culture developed around experiencing life near water.

Every summer our own little family makes a trek through the back roads of Michigan to my husband's favorite place in the world: the Kolber cottage at the lake. When we lived in Colorado, we sometimes flew through Chicago, but a few times we drove the sixteen-plus hours from Denver. We've honored births, deaths, birthdays, pregnancies, engagements, weddings, anniversaries, baptisms, Thanksgiving, Christmas, Memorial Day, Labor Day, the Fourth of July, and just about everything in between at that cottage. We've had sleepless nights with newborns there, had to coax our kids out of the water after too many hours in the sun there, and packed way too many people in a house there.

Before I met Brendan almost seventeen years ago, a friend of mine who wanted to set us up sent Brendan's work profile. The "get to know you" section included the question: "If you could travel anywhere, where would you go?"

His answer? To the lake, getting up right before the sun with a steaming cup of fresh coffee. Then, if possible, going out to water-ski at daybreak.

When we first married and began to take trips together to the Kolber cottage, I was introduced to the "crow's nest" (translation: a tiny triangle loft area above the living room that was just big enough for a mattress). This was where Brendan had slept for several years so he could be awakened by the first light in the morning. Now I was invited to join him in this small abode.

Bless our young hearts (not to mention our formerly strong backs)! That sleeping arrangement lasted only a few years as I needed a bit more rest than the tiny loft could provide.

We've lived a lot of life there on the shores of a small lake in Michigan. And every time we're there, Brendan comes alive. Honestly, once I sat next to the lake at sunset and saw Brendan's gigantic smile as the boat rounded a corner and he made a wide turn on his slalom ski, I could see why. So now whenever we go to the cottage, I don't think of it just as a place or a trip—I'm reminded that this is where Brendan connects with and embodies a vital glimmer of joy, making the trek worth it every time.[1]

FINDING THE GLIMMERS

Therapist Deb Dana coined the term *glimmer* to refer to experiences, sensations, or "micro moments" that cue safety, calm, or regulation in our nervous system.[2] In every respect, a glimmer is the opposite of what is often called a trigger. If a trigger is anything (smell, taste, experience, person, etc.) that activates an embodied memory of a past threat or trauma, a glimmer is something that helps us connect with a sense of our felt safety and step back into our window of tolerance (or, in polyvagal theory, our ventral vagal system). I love the language of glimmer because it literally speaks to *lighting up* a vital part of ourselves that makes us human. Tuning in to glimmers essentially makes us feel connected, curious, creative, compassionate, alive, and more.

Just about anything that lights up our ventral vagal can be a resource. Though the lake at Kolber cottage has become quite special to me, I've come to recognize that this is the place of about a million glimmers of goodness for Brendan. For Iris, having a reparative experience with her boss is now a significant glimmer for her.

Occasionally, in the middle of an already harried day, I will receive a text from my dear friend Ashley, who lives on the other side of the country. Basically she says something like this: "I have a ventral bomb for you. Check this out . . ." She will have sent me some sort of animal meme, a ridiculous GIF, or maybe even a parenting TikTok video. Inevitably, I will giggle pretty hard and confirm that she was right. She provided a ventral bomb that helped me tap into my true self: After seeing it, I feel lighter, my cheeks are a tiny bit red, and my heart feels much more open.

As we think about glimmers and resourcing, I invite you to consider this verse from Philippians 4:8: "Finally, brothers and sisters, whatever is true, whatever is noble, whatever is right, whatever is pure, whatever is lovely, whatever is admirable—if anything is excellent or praiseworthy—think about such things."

This verse is a powerful example of modeling both glimmers and resourcing for believers. It's vital we remember that we have a God who can hold and honor both our lament *and* our joy. We don't and shouldn't shame uncomfortable emotions (like sadness, anger, despair, confusion). We know we have a God who asks us to "weep with those who weep" (Romans 12:15, ESV). But as we look at the Philippians passage, we see that we are also invited to honor and cultivate emotions that bring us comfort. They're just as important. This verse *itself* offers a resource of what it might look like to allow our brains to be shaped by goodness, built on the ultimate resource: God with us.

Certainly—and this is an important disclaimer—for trauma survivors, goodness has at times been so fleeting and unavailable that initially, our bodies may feel triggered[3] or unable to fully savor something comforting. Without proper pacing of our nervous system, it may even feel overwhelming at first. But just like with all of our work, we can trust that God gave our bodies wisdom to help us know how to begin learning to experience these moments at the pace we are able.

A RESURRECTION HOPE

All glimmers and resources are reminders of the with-ness and witness of a God who loves us madly. My friend and fellow therapist Dr. Alison Cook compares the idea of glimmers to hope—not only in everyday life, but also as it's demonstrated in the Bible.[4] I happen to agree with her that whether goodness comes through common or specific grace, it is a form of tangible hope. And as the apostle Paul writes in Romans 5:3, we can glory in (not because of) our suffering; knowing that because God is with us, God can cause even those things that have harmed us to help develop our endurance, character, and hope. And here's possibly my favorite part: *This hope* does not put us to shame (5:5).

Paul points to this paradoxical hope—this strength like water that becomes embedded in the core of who we are—when he writes: "We are hard pressed on every side, but not crushed; perplexed, but not in despair; persecuted, but not abandoned; struck down, but not destroyed. We always carry around in our body the death of Jesus, so that the life of Jesus may also be revealed in *our body*" (2 Corinthians 4:8-10, emphasis mine). When Paul speaks about the death of Jesus, perhaps he is pointing to the fact that Jesus' willingness to come for us and to sacrifice Himself for us is profound evidence of our belovedness. I love the phrasing "we always carry around in our body" because we now understand that we carry trauma and pain in our body like a story.

How fitting, then, that we are invited to *carry around in our bodies* a love that does not disappoint or put us to shame.

This is how we come alive. As my friend and fellow therapist Ryan Kuja writes, "Resurrection is in our cells."[5] Every time we help our body feel safe, we are practicing hope and resurrection. Every time we turn with compassion to ourselves and others, we, as Wendell Berry says, "Practice resurrection."[6] Every time we feel the sun on our cheeks and the wind in our hair and the breath in our lungs; when we laugh at a joke or feel the embrace of people who love us, we are practicing the brave work of resurrection. In a world where there is much pain and destruction, seeing resurrection is no small thing.

STRENGTHENING THE RESOURCE

Attention itself can help to anchor a resource in our bodies, but I have learned an additional way to support folks as well. As a therapist trained in EMDR (eye movement desensitization and reprocessing), I help clients unlock previously "stuck" disturbances[7] they have held in their bodies. EMDR facilitates healing by allowing both sides of our brain to work together in order for trauma memories to be influenced and adapted by newer, resourced ones.[8] When this occurs, the more resourced memories or experiences help to increase our window of tolerance, thereby bringing the systems of the body that can "digest" the trauma back online—and this ultimately allows disturbing memories to fully process through our bodies.

One of the main methods used in EMDR to support folks as they process trauma is through the use of bilateral stimulation (BLS).[9] It sounds super clinical, but really, bilateral stimulation is any type of rhythmic "alternating right, left stimulation,"[10] whether touch, sound, or eye movements. For example, over the course of the pandemic I have done much more teletherapy.

During these sessions, I often invite clients to self tap during an EMDR or resourcing session either by crossing their arms over their chests and alternate tapping on their shoulders (sometimes called butterfly tapping), or I will invite them to rest their hands on their legs and tap in an alternating fashion. In the case of EMDR, trained therapists can utilize a specific protocol to help clients process trauma. But importantly, this practice is not confined just to the therapeutic world. Anytime we take a walk, or swing our arms, or dance, or look side to side, we are using bilateral stimulation. For me personally, walking (and occasionally jogging) has become a vital lifeline to my mental health and resourcing. Engaging in one of these activities while enjoying life-giving music or natural beauty allows my body to have a higher capacity to process and receive the goodness that's available. That's why I often pair a few worship songs or guided meditations with my exercise: I know I will feel even more grounded afterward. Dr. Laurel Parnell refers to this as "resource tapping" or "tapping in."[11] It's a way to internalize a resource so that neural pathways connect it to our full brain, making it more accessible when we are in our window of tolerance.

As we build up and strengthen our resources, we are creating more and more felt safety in our bodies. For those of us who have experienced a severe and chronic lack of safety, this work is especially important. People who have had experiences of "good enough parenting" and "good enough safety" will discover that their bodies will intuitively be more likely to reach for resourcing in moments of difficulty. But learning to resource is a helpful and important practice to support the flourishing of any person.

In some ways, tapping into a resource is a little like turning up music. If you feel generally comforted by a resource or an experience, it's as if your speaker is turned up to a 4 out of 10. It's pleasant but soft enough that it's still easy to get distracted from it—maybe you don't hear the words and miss some details. But if you tap into that resource with some bilateral stimulation, you've turned the volume up to a 7, 8, or sometimes even a 10. Now the music and words are clearer. Bilateral stimulation helps make us more present and accessible to resources, which we can experience in a richer and deeper way.[12]

Reader, I'd like to pause for a moment with you and just celebrate what this means. Even when life is profoundly hard, we are invited to partake, as we're able, in goodness. I've written in the past that God is a keeper and curator of our stories. And every single part of those stories matters. Not only that, but there is a beautiful mystery that allows the painful experiences we've weathered using situational strength to be transformed so we can move toward a deeper, fuller, and more integrated strength. This reflects what our God is like—with us, always; working for, in, and through even the most dire of circumstances, always.

THE GOD WHO RESOURCES US

Recently, I'd been experiencing a situation that had many pitfalls and discouragements. While walking the hills by our house one day, I called my sister, Steph, and told her about its many twists and turns. For a moment, she was quiet.

"Would it be okay if I shared something I feel like God is reminding me?" she asked.

"Sure," I said, curious.

And then she told me how God had been meeting her recently with these words from Scripture: "Put on the full armor of God, so that . . . you may be able to stand your ground, and after you have done everything, to stand. Stand firm then" (Ephesians 6:13-14).

"Do you hear it, Aundi?" she asked me. "Do you hear the invitation?"

Something in me lit up when I recognized God's encouragement that, after we've done everything, we should stand.

How do we do that, God? I wondered. *How do we stand when we're exhausted, afraid, or just plain sad? How do we keep going?*

And then a few weeks later, I got it—as my feet hit the pavement on another walk. When the writer of Ephesians tells the reader to put on "the full armor of God," he is inviting us to compassionately resource ourselves, to become strong like water. When we have the safety of God's connection to us paired with the resources named in Ephesians 6:14-15—God's truth, righteousness, and peace—we can navigate hardship, pain, and evil differently. Our good God recognizes that in order to truly navigate everything that may come our way, we are going to need resources. We are going to need His good gifts.

It's not as if I hadn't heard or read Ephesians 6 before my sister reminded me of this passage. But bringing the lens of polyvagal theory, interpersonal neurobiology, and attachment transforms how I read that Scripture now. God knows how we are created. He knows we can't simply spiritually bypass our way into putting on this different type of armor. God knows we can only authentically access resources and participate when we feel safe enough to do so.

That is an important nuance in our discussion. If we face external factors—such as the ongoing systemic trauma of poverty, discrimination, or racism—we will likely have more difficulty accessing resources. This is so, so valid (and by God's grace, we will continue to correct injustice). But though we may be limited in what we can change, we can still leverage what *is* available now—even if that is only the knowledge that a past traumatic event was neither okay nor our fault and that it's now over. Working to release shame and reminding ourselves that we are beloved survivors can in and of itself be an empowering resource.

Perhaps this is why God constantly reminds us that He is "close to the brokenhearted" and "saves those who are crushed in spirit" (Psalm 34:18). While recognizing that we are so very human and will fall short, we can hold that truth in tension with His invitation to think on "whatever is true, whatever is noble, whatever is right, whatever is pure, whatever is lovely, whatever is admirable—if anything is excellent or praiseworthy—think about such things" (Philippians 4:8).

Our humanity doesn't surprise God. Our need for connection, safety, and authenticity doesn't in any way dishonor God—because that's how we were designed. As Jesus said, "In this world you will have trouble. But take heart! I have overcome the world" (John 16:33). Jesus knew, my friends. He isn't surprised when we are struggling, and yet our God is with us, inviting us to flow toward healing and wholeness.

BECOMING STRONG LIKE WATER

Resources are essential if we are to internalize a sense of safety. One beautiful thing about the way God designed our bodies is that we don't have to have everything figured out or all our wounds healed to begin the journey of resourcing. Even though we are limited and fragile, our bodies can change and grow. What a miracle.

In this section, inspired by the work of Dr. Laurel Parnell,[13] you will assess the resources in your life so that you are better able to leverage what may already be available to you. If you aren't able to fill in all the following exercises at once, that's okay. Additionally, as it feels supportive to you, you may add in tapping (or other types of bilateral stimulation) to the resources below. Generally, when you add in tapping to a resource, I recommend bringing that resource into your mind's eye and then noticing any supportive sensations that accompany it. For example, you might describe the resource through sight, smell, touch, hearing, and/or taste (if applicable). You may wish to use the somatic vocabulary on page 147 to help support you in this.

Next, as you think on the resource, tap for fifteen to twenty seconds at a time. For example, as you visualize a beautiful sunset, you might close your eyes and use your fingertips to alternate tapping on your right and left knees. Doing so will help connect that resource to neural pathways on both sides of your brain. If possible, do this at least three times to help strengthen these neural pathways, each time noticing if the resource itself is becoming more anchored in your body. Feel free to complete the section below as you're able:

RELATIONAL RESOURCES[14]

Is there a particular person who has helped you feel calm or safe? If so, I invite you to describe details such as who they are, how they communicate with you, how you feel when you're with them, and any other characteristics that feel supportive to you; e.g., are they protective, nurturing, kind? (Note: It's okay if you can't come up with someone.)

Do you have a memory of feeling cared for? If yes, briefly write it out below. (Note: It's okay if you can't come up with a memory.)

Somatic Vocabulary

An important part of moving trauma and stress through your body is learning to tune in and describe your bodily sensations.[15] Once you do so, you can decide how to move or otherwise support your body so that the feeling doesn't remain stuck inside you.

This vocabulary list might be a good starting point for you, but I encourage you to remain curious and add your own words as you learn to attune to the sensations of your body.

Achy	Open
Airy	Pointy
Anchored	Prickly
Buzzy	Pulsing
Clear	Radiating
Cold	Rough
Contracted	Satiated
Electric	Saturated
Expansive	Small
Full	Smooth
Fuzzy	Soggy
Grounded	Tender
Hard	Tense
Heavy	Tight
Hot	Tingly
Light	Trembling
Loose	Vibrating
Lukewarm	Wobbly

If it is hard to come up with real-life examples for either of these first two questions (which is common for those who've experienced attachment wounding or trauma), take a moment to consider if there is a character from a book, movie, or even your imagination that you can envision feeling comfortable around or making you feel cared for. If so, take a moment and write out who the character is and what they're like.

PHYSICAL RESOURCES

Is there a place (in nature or elsewhere) where you have felt calm, safe, or protected? If so, I invite you to write about that place briefly below. Please share as much sensory information as feels helpful as you consider this place (e.g., what you would see, smell, hear if you were there).

If there is not an actual place in your life where you have felt consistently safe (common among survivors of trauma), is there an imaginary place where you can imagine feeling calm, safe, or protected? This can truly be wherever you would like. Again, share as much sensory information as possible as you consider this place.

BOUNDARY RESOURCES

Can you recall a time in your life when you have been able to say no or set a boundary? If this is a challenge for you, you may choose to think of someone in your life who you believe sets boundaries in a way you would like to embody. If this resource feels flooding at this time, you may always choose to pass. However, if you can recall either an experience in your own life or someone you've observed—even for something that may seem unimportant—please take a moment to write about it and why it felt empowering.

SPIRITUAL RESOURCES

Do you experience your faith as a resource? For many the answer is yes, but unfortunately for those who have experienced abuse or mistreatment in church or another faith community, this may not be true. As always, please utilize this section to the extent that it feels helpful, knowing that God's posture toward you remains kind. Please feel free to adapt the prompts below or discontinue them if they don't feel like a useful resource.

In this section, take a moment to recall a time when you felt connected to God. What was happening in your life? As you reflect on this, what do you notice in your body?

Is there a particular Scripture(s), hymn, and/or song that helps you feel connected to God? If so, list them below.

Is there a person who reminds you of what Jesus is like? If so, explain.

Is there any other spiritual experience that feels important to add here? If so, feel free to write about it.

OBJECTS AS RESOURCES

Do you have any tangible items that may be a resource to you? For example, I love books, candles (including battery-operated ones), soft and heavy blankets, and my favorite sweatshirt. Describe anything that comes to mind below.

EXPERIENCES AS RESOURCES

As you are able, describe a time when you felt empowered:

As you are able, describe a time you felt capable:

As you are able, describe a time you were able to try something new:

As you are able, describe an experience that surprised you when it turned out better than planned:

To the extent that it feels supportive, I invite you to return to these touch points in the future.

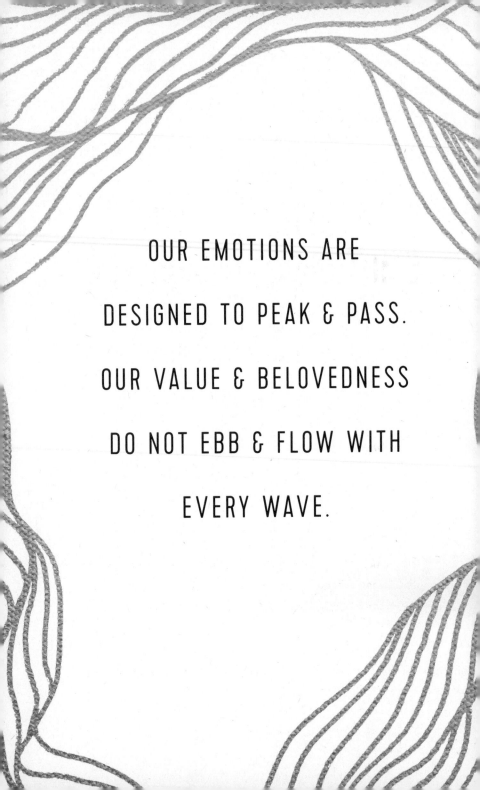

OUR EMOTIONS ARE

DESIGNED TO PEAK & PASS.

OUR VALUE & BELOVEDNESS

DO NOT EBB & FLOW WITH

EVERY WAVE.

CHAPTER 7

STRENGTH WITH EMOTIONAL FLEXIBILITY

You can't stop the waves, but you can learn to surf.
JON KABAT-ZINN

Crying does not indicate that you are weak. Since birth,
it has always been a sign that you are alive.
ATTRIBUTED TO CHARLOTTE BRONTË

WHEN TIARA AND I FIRST WORKED TOGETHER a few years ago, she realized that her story held much unresolved relational and attachment trauma from her childhood. We'd begun helping Tiara build safety and resources, but when life got busy and full for her, we needed to pause our work. Such is life.

In the interim, Tiara married and later struggled with

infertility. Then, about a year after that, Tiara called to get back into counseling after she and her husband lost their home in a fire. The panic attacks and bad dreams she thought she'd put behind her had returned with a vengeance.

"I suppose I thought healing meant I wouldn't feel quite so much," she told me. "Several people from our faith community were supportive right after the fire. They even helped us replace many of the items we'd lost. It was honestly so helpful. But then it felt like a switch was flipped. People started to imply that we just needed more faith to deal with losing our house.

"Even though I tried to act fine and be on my best behavior, sometimes I would find myself crying in church because I couldn't hold it all in. Suddenly I felt so much shame about not being 'over it' yet."

One Sunday, Tiara told me, was particularly devastating. Their pastor, who was preaching a series on conquering feelings, told the story of a couple from his former church whose home had gone into foreclosure after both lost their jobs. Rather than falling into despair, the pastor said, the couple moved in with the wife's parents, who needed help maintaining their property anyway. "That couple didn't give *up*; they gave *out* of what they still had!" the pastor boomed.

After the service, someone from Tiara's small group came up to her. Putting a hand on Tiara's arm, the woman said, "I think that sermon was just for you! See, God will work everything out for your good. There's always a silver lining if you just look hard enough!" Seeing another friend, this woman smiled and just walked away. Instead of reminding Tiara that Jesus was right there with her as she grieved and lamented, this woman left Tiara feeling shunned.

"I thought that if I appeared self-composed, it was proof that I was further along in my spiritual journey," Tiara said with a heavy sigh. "I thought I shouldn't show any emotion because, in my head, that somehow equated to being 'stronger' or 'more faithful.' I think I've been doing this same thing my whole life. I've always been such a deep feeler, but honestly, I don't think many people can handle that."

I let Tiara's words hang for a moment as I considered my reply. Her unprocessed grief and suppressed emotion were palpable.

"What has that been like for you, Tiara?" I asked.

"Terrible, honestly. Lonely. But what other choice do I have? I don't know another way," she said.

At first, Tiara had tried to navigate the fire like all the other pain in her life: by either completely pushing it down or feeling it intensely for a moment in private and then shaming herself afterward. *Who do I think I am*, she would ask herself, *thinking I can let myself fall apart like that?*

And when members of her church seemed to confirm the idea that her faith was at the center of her suffering, something in her broke.

She looked at me with tears in her eyes. "This can't be what God is actually like, can it?"

Tiara's situational strength worked until it didn't. Initially, we worked on reestablishing her sense of safety and building up some of her resources. The persistent panic attacks and nightmares, she realized, were ways her body was trying to communicate a message to her: Engaging in this type of spiritual bypassing was not only unhelpful, it was harmful.

She and her husband began to prayerfully consider their next steps. Though it took some time to find ways to rebuild safety, they eventually transitioned to a different faith community that honored and acknowledged their grief. Little by little, Tiara began to learn gentle ways to feel her emotions. God didn't want her to stuff her emotions. He wanted her to feel the whole spectrum of them, just as Jesus did.

Filled with feeling—that's what God was really like.

THE INVALUABLE INFORMATION OF EMOTIONS

We can suppress, shame, and numb our emotions for only so long. To survive, Tiara had been required to draw on situational strength such as repressing and spiritual bypassing for much of her life. She simply didn't have the safety needed to move toward a more integrated strength. And, as I reminded her, that was totally valid. There's no shame in surviving.

But God designed us not just to survive, but to thrive. As

we discussed in *Try Softer*, emotions give us clues as to what's happening in our bodies, our psyches, and sometimes our spirits. When we view emotions this way rather than through a shame-based lens (that they are either good or bad), we are more likely to see our emotions as keys to integration, wholeness, and the honoring of our full humanity. They can guide us to what we truly need. And as we gain resources and support, we can learn to honor the reality that our emotions are designed to peak and pass. Our value and belovedness do not ebb and flow with every wave. Instead, those waves simply provide information.

Like Tiara, many of us learned early that we couldn't ride those waves, perhaps because those emotional currents contained information that felt too overwhelming and disturbing to our bodies. As a result, we used situational strength to build armor around the pain. Healing looks like compassionately *turning toward* difficult experiences—and providing resources that communicate to our bodies that it's safe to feel what we feel. Learning to work with our own nervous system (sometimes with the support of a therapist) will help us become attuned to what we need through the process.

Generally, what we feel in any given moment is based on three possibilities: We could be feeling an emotion because of an unprocessed event in our past that has been activated; it could be that the emotion is based solely in the present moment; or it could be a combination of the two. It's important to remain open and curious about where the emotion we are experiencing is based; otherwise, our emotions are likely to remain intensified. They're telling us what they need—and if we don't listen, they're going to get louder.

If we think our feelings are *always* only about past trauma, we may miss important information from the present that can help us meet a need or stop harm. For example, Tiara's childhood trauma certainly affected how she was processing the loss of her house to a fire. Yet the messages of spiritual bypassing from her faith community in the present were *also* affecting her. On the other hand, if we think our emotions are *exclusively* about the present, we may miss valuable information about how we can continue to heal. That's why validating Tiara's present circumstances mattered, but so did remaining attuned to the way her past set her up to believe that her only option was to suppress her emotions. Once she understood this, she could use compassion and curiosity to navigate the important information her body offered her. She could then remain open and attuned to respond as needed.

A FLEXIBLE DANCE

So what might it look like to compassionately resource emotions?

When I teach my clients about this concept, I love to use the metaphor of dance. The hip-hop artist, ballerina, and tap dancer display tremendous physical artistry, but in fact,

God made all of our bodies to learn to *move with* what we're experiencing.

When I think about the way we were designed to process life's experiences, I absolutely love the observation, generally attributed to Ram Dass, that "you can do it like it's a great weight on you, or you can do it like a dance." At our best, I believe this is what we are made for. And yet, dancing has never been an option for many of us, even when we wanted it to be. When we experience trauma or hold emotional disturbances in our body, our movements become limited. Such pain creates rigidity (hyperarousal) or, in some cases, a sense of complete collapse (hypoarousal). Of course, neither tightly bound rigidity nor breakdown serves us well in a dance. Movement *requires* flexibility, and many dancers work and practice developing this skill.

Similarly, a rigid approach to our inner world can inhibit us from feeling emotions in the way we need. A part of becoming strong like water is learning to be *emotionally flexible*.[1] As we learn to dance *with* our pain and discomfort, we become able to "weep with those who weep" (Romans 12:15, ESV) while also honoring and experiencing "inexpressible and glorious joy" (1 Peter 1:8, NIV). We enlarge our capacity to be human and offer our "with-ness" to others too.

So let's put on our dancing shoes.

Learn the basics

Like almost everything we do, learning to increase emotional flexibility begins in the body. In a quite simplistic way, we think about emotion as energy that mobilizes because something needs attention (e-motion).[2] With this lens, we can learn to (1) pay attention to a sensation; (2) ride the wave of the emotion; (3) respond appropriately to it; (4) name the emotion as it feels helpful; (5) allow it to dissipate; and (6) if the emotion is too big to be felt all at once, practice grounding or containment and come back to it.[3]

Additionally, as we become more adept at processing emotion, we realize that not everything we feel will require a major response but often better aligns with small and attuned responses over time. For example, my client Sam found that as he learned to listen, attune, and compassionately resource his body in our sessions, his emotional flexibility grew. He began to intuitively know that his body was capable of moving through feelings rather than remaining stuck in them. Additionally, Sam came to realize that by simply noticing body sensations and allowing them to peak and pass, he was able to process his experiences, listening to his emotions without allowing them to dictate everything he did.

Increase your emodiversity

In 2014, researchers conducted a study to examine *emodiversity*, or experiencing a balance of both pleasant and uncomfortable emotions. The researchers discovered something that seems paradoxical but is quite helpful in our strong-like-water work. Essentially, a greater diversity of positive and negative emotions correlates with lower experiences of depression and higher overall well-being.

Researchers can't say exactly why this is the case, but this is their theory:

> [Just as] biodiversity increases resilience to negative events because a single predator cannot wipe out an entire ecosystem, emodiversity may prevent specific emotions—in particular detrimental ones such as acute stress, anger or sadness—from dominating the emotional ecosystem. For instance, the experience of prolonged sadness might lead to depression but *the joint experience of sadness and anger—although unpleasant—might prevent individuals from completely withdrawing from their environment.* The same biodiversity analogy could be applied to positive emotion. Humans are notoriously quick to adapt to repeated exposure to a given positive emotional experience; positive experiences that are diverse may be more resistant to such extinction.[4]

Why does this matter for us? As we learn to experience the full range of our emotions, we are *stronger and more resilient*, not weaker. Certainly, we want to ensure that we have healthy doses of joy, compassion, excitement, and love in the mix—but not at the expense of honoring our full humanity.

WHEN THE EMOTION FEELS TOO BIG

One idea I commonly run into with trauma survivors—and truly with almost every person who has lived through the last several years—is that emotions are sometimes too big to be felt all at once. This was true for my client Erica, who often aspired to process everything she was feeling all at once just to get it over with. Erica had grown up with a father in the military who had unwittingly communicated that she was way too much for everyone, including him. Erica had brought this attachment trauma with her into an abusive marriage, which finally ended a few years ago—but not without leaving deep emotional scars.

In my work with Erica, I first taught her grounding and containment as options when something felt as if it would flood her nervous system. However, as our work continued, I also taught her additional ways to continue building her emotional flexibility.

Titration[5]

Whenever Erica began to dive into her history of trauma, I watched as she began to speak rapidly and her body tensed up. I could feel a sense of electricity in the room. Early on, I told Erica that she didn't need to share all her history or stories until she felt ready.[6] This strategy of easing in or taking something in smaller chunks is called *titration*.[7]

Whether you are working on your own or with a therapist, titration is a strategy you can apply to emotional processing or any experience or sensation that is bigger than you feel you can handle. In a way, just in making a disturbing topic/emotion/sensation/task smaller, you are compassionately resourcing yourself so that you can move along the flow of strength.

Pendulation[8]

Like titration, this next strategy also expands our tolerance for discomfort by carefully moving into something overwhelming and/or triggering. However, with *pendulation*, we begin by establishing a resource. Next, we ease into the discomfort of a disturbing event, memory, or emotion by pairing it with the already established resource. Then finally we "set down" the disturbance and end with connecting only to the resource. I like to think of it like the swinging pendulum of a grandfather clock. On one side of the pendulation we hold on to the resource; on the other we hold both the resource and the disturbance—and we swing between the two sides at the pace we need.

For example, Erica realized that flying had become triggering for her once the pandemic began. To help Erica with this, we first firmly established a grounding resource: a memory of a time when Erica did something brave by trying a cooking class that she felt slightly terrified about but that she ended up loving. This resource helped expand Erica's window of tolerance so she could remain open to the idea of flying. Erica told me that the memory of the cooking class brought to the forefront that though flying felt scary, she also knew that not everything that feels overwhelming leads to actual danger. It helped her remember that sometimes being brave leads to new opportunities and adventure—and this helped Erica find a way through her anxiety.

When I guided her through pendulation, Erica "brought" the resource with her while taking a moment to shift her focus to the thought of flying—and the pit in her stomach that accompanied that thought. When Erica paired the cooking class memory with the thought of flying, it didn't magically get easier—but it was as though the supportive memory was an added resource; it softened the fear by helping her remember that she had done hard things before. Once she was comfortable, Erica attempted to "set down" thinking about flying, and she finished by connecting only to the resource.

This strategy may seem counterintuitive and complex, but it was highly helpful for Erica as she continued to build her emotional flexibility. By pendulating her focus, she was able to stay within—and even expand—her window of tolerance while also strengthening her ability to move through and process her hard experience.[9]

THE EDGE WHERE IT HAPPENS

It can feel like a difficult truth, but it's truth just the same: The edges of our discomfort are where significant growth happens. And certainly we always hold this tension with the reality that many of us trauma survivors have lived most of our lives outside our comfort zone or on the edges. This is why we always build safety and support before we even consider navigating to the edge. Prior to encouraging you to risk something, I want to make sure you have a soft place to land. Remember when we discussed the idea of discomfort versus harm in chapter 2? We always want to do our best to stay in the zone of discomfort—not harm—in this work.

However, when we view this idea through the lens of our window of tolerance, it is only when we take the risk of putting one foot *outside* our window (keeping the other foot safely and firmly planted inside it) that we have the opportunity to *expand* our window. From a neurobiological perspective, this nervous system straddling is called a *blended state* or *mixed state*.[10] Blended states are where the magic happens when it comes to emotional flexibility—when we grow our window, we grow our flexibility. There is potential in these blended states for great reward as our bodies learn to expand into healing—but there is also potential for great harm if we aren't keenly attuned to our own needs and limits.

Dr. Arielle Schwartz describes the practice and process of expanding our tolerance like this:

This involves initially developing your capacity to feel peaceful, calm, and connected. Once you have a solid foundation of being able to access your social nervous system you can slowly build your tolerance for distressing physiological activation. This is

accomplished by blending social engagement with
both mobilization and immobilization until you
can re-establish a sense of safety with those nervous
system states. Over time, you increase your capacity
to move in and out of different nervous system
states.[11]

Dr. Schwartz is describing the trajectory of our strong-like-
water work. We establish safety: We seek experiences of care
and goodness; we come to know that we are loved. We then
begin to play, becoming acquainted with the joy of movement for fun and recreation (mobilization) as well as the
serenity that can come with simply taking in beauty and
goodness while being still (immobilization). Little by little,
our window grows. We become able to sit with a spectrum
of emotions, to recognize when we need more support, to
express our needs and desires to trusted loved ones.

Many folks were given such opportunities at young
ages and throughout their childhood. But a lack of safety,
or various types of harm, oppression, discrimination, poverty, racism, trauma, or toxic stress[12] kept many of us from
developing the internal frameworks we need to move beyond
situational strength and flow toward a growth edge—to flow
into a blended state. This is why, especially for trauma survivors, but truly for every human—learning about our nervous
system and these growth edges or blended states matters.
When discomfort always equals emergency, we never feel safe
enough to take that risk.

STRENGTH AND NEUROBIOLOGY

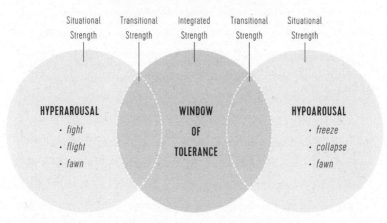

It's by learning to exist in this space of blended states that we can truly appreciate and leverage the connection with—truly *be with*—those we love and the God who loves us. It enables us to come alongside the younger parts of ourselves in the place of a loving parent as well. But also—and this especially excites me—this is where we can lovingly leverage the resources we begin to acquire when our bodies move into a sympathetic or parasympathetic state.

The *with-ness* is the medicine.

KEEPING ONE FOOT IN THE WINDOW

As you look to practice blended states and thereby increase your emotional flexibility, I encourage you to remember that we try to keep "one foot" in our window of tolerance.[13] In EMDR reprocessing, this type of psychological posture is called dual awareness,[14] and it's an absolute necessity whenever we process disturbing or overwhelming emotions. While we are not necessarily doing trauma processing here, please be aware you may need a therapist to support you if you find you don't yet have the capacity to hold this dual awareness on your own.

And as always, *there is no shame in this*—it's totally normal to need additional support at various times, even for experiences that may not feel challenging to others. You might also consider practicing with something that feels less disturbing (e.g., how you feel when you're running late or your friend forgets to call you back) to begin building up your capacity. But however you do it, building your tolerance for these blended states is an important part of the journey.

You may be ready to experience a blended state if you feel:

- an ability to say "I am noticing that . . ." or "I am aware I'm feeling . . ."; this mindful language is also a way you can engage your prefrontal cortex and stay in your WOT
- a sense that though a disturbing or traumatic memory still has a charge, it is not happening in the present
- an awareness of being connected to your body

The following practices, inspired by the work of Dr. Arielle Schwartz,[15] are ways you might get curious about what blended states feel like, and how you can experience them.

Ventral Vagal/Window of Tolerance

Before we can understand what it's like to experience a blended state, we need to remember what it feels like when you are firmly within your window of tolerance. You might notice that you feel open to connection and relationship, which has the potential to be one of our greatest resources. Additionally, you may feel available to new experiences, a sense that you are capable, a capacity to be flexible in the face of challenges, an openness to God, and more. I love how the Internal Family Systems[16] model recognizes that when someone is connected to their core "Self" (or, as I think of it, grounded in their WOT), they may experience connection with what authors and therapists Alison Cook and Kimberly Miller call your Spirit-led self. Cook and Miller note that qualities such as calmness, clarity, curiosity, compassion, confidence, courage, creativity, and connectivity are often the product of this Self.[17]

As we begin this work, I recommend finding or creating a resource(s) that helps you feel solidly in your WOT. (Refer back to chapter 6 if needed.) I also recommend identifying one supportive resource you can access when you experience hyperarousal and one you can use when you are in hypoarousal. This will help you be able to quickly step back into your WOT if your nervous system becomes overwhelmed as you move toward the blended state.

Safe Mobilization (sympathetic nervous system blended with window of tolerance[18])

Think of the difference between running from a tiger versus running because we're playing a game of tag. One is based on survival and the other is based on play. Safe mobilization is the latter; our body might be working hard, but it's in service of movement, play, and even wholeness. In safe mobilization, it's as though we have one foot connected to our sympathetic nervous system (which focuses on mobilizing us) and one foot in our WOT (also known as our ventral vagal complex). Safe mobilization looks like helping our body truly integrate the reality that we *are* safe even while accessing movement. For those of us whose bodies had to learn to live in a braced state, constantly hypervigilant and going into fight, flight, or potentially fawn mode at any potential danger, our experience may tell us that it's safe not to do anything.

To practice safe mobilization, consider first using one of the various resources we have already established (grounding, containment, orienting, reparenting statements, etc.). Once you've done that, ease into some movement (dance, run, jump).

Next, pause to notice that it is safe to move in this way.

Take a moment going back and forth between these practices and see if you can bring the safety "with you" as you mobilize.

Safe Immobilization (dorsal vagal complex blended with window of tolerance[19])

For many of us who've experienced trauma, feeling trapped or immobilized has been part of what has felt so overwhelming.

Thus, for many of us, anything that reminds us of a sense of being trapped can be triggering—even experiences of stillness that are in actuality safe. In response to this, we may find ourselves constantly in motion, never letting ourselves settle because even subconsciously this may be experienced as a threat. Over time, this inability to feel safe while calm or still can be profoundly harmful to us, even though at one point it likely kept us safe.

Similar to safe mobilization, our work here is to have a tether, or one foot inside of our WOT while still accessing a bit of our dorsal vagal in order to access a blended state of calm, stillness, or intimacy. In other words, utilizing our social engagement system (i.e., remaining in our window of tolerance) keeps our bodies from heading into fawn/freeze or collapse when we want to experience stillness in a way that feels safe to our bodies.[20]

To practice safe immobilization, first consider using one of the various resources we have already established (grounding, containment, orienting, reparenting statements, etc.). Once you've done that, ease into some stillness (standing, sitting, lying). As you do this, observe your body and your breath; pause to notice that it is safe to be still. Feel free to make this practice as short as needed, knowing that over time as you mindfully engage this work, your tolerance will grow.

WHEN GRIEVING GROWS US

During these last few years, I've thought about grief often. Perhaps because there has been so much to grieve in a world that seems to be falling apart at the seams. But the truth is, I've always been well acquainted with grief. I think that's why I am often so attracted to Jesus, "a man of sorrows" (Isaiah 53:3, NLT). So many people hid their faces from Him because He was so acquainted with grief, yet I see this aspect of Him as a profound expression of God with us.

In fact, I have to tell you that as someone who has experienced my fair share of folks wanting to put a nice, tidy bow on my story, knowing that Jesus was deeply connected to grief heartens me in a way that is beyond words and brings me great courage in my work as both a therapist and a survivor of trauma.

In her famous poem "The Hill We Climb," national youth poet laureate Amanda Gorman writes, "That even as we grieved, we grew."[21] The first time I heard that poem, my heart resounded within me. I knew exactly what she meant. I certainly don't enjoy grieving, and yet there is something sacred about it.

The Bible calls the practice of grieving lamenting. And I love the practice-based element to lament because grieving is more than an idea. It's an embodied way of expressing and releasing our deep pain. Perhaps this is why actions such as repenting with sackcloth and ashes (Job 42:6; Lamentations 2:10; Luke 10:13) and wailing (Jeremiah 9:17-26) are key elements of the Old Testament; they model a sacred engagement with God while in pain. Theologian Soong-Chan Rah notes, "The hope of lament is that God would respond to human suffering that is wholeheartedly communicated through lament."[22] Lament, in particular, is a way of expressing our grief to God, while knowing we are held.

Why does this matter so much? As renowned psychiatrist Gabor Maté writes, "Genuine grieving is the opposite of trauma."[23] And if grief is part of what it means to be human, an inability to grieve is costly. Some of us may have suppressed our ability to grieve as a means of survival—we may feel that we didn't have a choice. This is the beautiful work of becoming flexible with our emotions, of working to truly acknowledge and allowing ourselves to feel our reality. It's the work of a lifetime, and it is a holy endeavor.

And as we learn to grieve, we are held by our Creator. Maybe that's why Henri Nouwen's observation that "I am beginning to see that much of praying is grieving" strikes me differently now.[24] If God calls us to "pray without ceasing" (1 Thessalonians 5:17, ESV), could it be that as we learn to abide and exist within God, He is constantly holding us as we feel and pray? It seems to me that Nouwen had identified an element of true strength: When God holds us in our pain, we have access to an abundant resource that allows us to be fully human. As we learn to accept our grief, we become more and more able to remain present to our human experience. We are no longer permanently stuck outside of our window of tolerance—constantly operating out of situational strength.

God is with us. God does hold us, even when we don't know it. Even when we can't hold on to God, God holds on to us.

And this is one of the mysteries of grief; this sacred space where we allow our pain to be tended and honored is, as Gabor Maté says, the opposite of trauma.

This is why, even though it may seem counterintuitive, I invite you to see how grief—allowing ourselves to feel our painful feelings in a way that is tolerable to our bodies—is a core part of becoming strong like water.

It's only when we have the ability to feel that we can also heal.

BECOMING STRONG LIKE WATER: DANCING WITH HARD THINGS

For this resource, you may consider pulling out a journal to answer these questions.

When approaching a moment, emotion,[25] conversation, or event that might feel difficult or overwhelming, one phenomenal place to begin is to ask ourselves this simple question:

What kind of support would I need to do _____?

For many of us, it's not intuitive to ask this question—the only option we've ever had is to live from the survival energy of situational strength. But learning to move along the flow of strength gives us freedom to do things differently.

For example, let's go back to the story of Tiffany from chapter 1. One practice she began was to identify her resources, not just generally, but specifically.

When Tiffany knew she was going to have a challenging conversation with her mother, we took time in a session to think through and then practice what she would need to stay connected to her window of tolerance as she visited with her mom.

Initially she joked, "Aundi, I don't think this is what you mean, but in order for me to have this conversation with my mom, she will need to start therapy in the next twenty-four hours."

Alas, don't all of us sometimes desire to control that which is outside our control? It would make things so easy. Unfortunately, Tiffany's mom had told her she wasn't open to additional support at this point. For Tiffany to pin her success or failure on what her mom did or didn't do would not ultimately help her as she learned to navigate her own story.

So then I reframed the question: "Based on what is actually in *your* control, what support would you need to be able to have this conversation?"

"Oh, that's a good question—but a tough one. I guess I would need to remember that I'm an adult now. If my mom begins to act in a way that is disrespectful or feels unsafe, I don't even need to have this conversation with her. Success for me in this situation would be setting the limits I need to feel safe, even if that means I need to actually leave," Tiffany replied, followed by a big exhale.

I paused, noticing the shift she was beginning to experience. "As you tell me those things, what are you noticing in your body?" I asked.

"I feel . . . extremely present and clear. I also sense a good tingling, especially in my chest and neck. Like I can hold my head up," she answered.

Next, I introduced the concept of a *future video* to Tiffany. This is a form of visualization—essentially, you run a "video" of the potential challenge in your mind's eye while *simultaneously* employing resources to keep you tethered to safety.[26] Tiffany and I listed several resources that she could "bring

Try *Softer* Language[27]

- What is the gentlest thing I could do today?
- What words or affirmations remind me of my true self?
- I wonder if I could take this in smaller steps?
- What would help me stay in my window of tolerance?
- What kind of support do I need to make this happen?
- Whom could I reach out to if I'm feeling overwhelmed?
- How could I help my body feel safe right now?
- What part of myself needs support right now?
- What activity would be soothing for me when I'm feeling triggered?
- Is there a way I could move my body to help me feel more connected to myself?

with her" into the visualization to help her navigate the difficult conversation. As she ran this "video" of the difficult conversation she would have with her mom, she "watched" herself doing grounding right before she walked into the door to her mom's house. She also "saw" herself saying the mantras, "I have choices" and "It's okay to speak up" as she sat down at her mom's kitchen table. This would help center her and give her courage ahead of the conversation.

And then Tiffany envisioned her mom's body language as Tiffany began to tell her she wasn't comfortable being treated the way she had been. In this moment, Tiffany brought in a visualization of a bubble of light surrounding her so that she felt even more separate from her mom.

This was Tiffany's future video.

Tiffany and I ran this "video" three separate times, and each time we did, Tiffany noticed this imagined encounter got a little easier. The key was making sure she had enough resources so that her body felt safe enough to visualize it without becoming overly triggered. As I explained it to her, the process is a bit like dipping your big toe into cold water. You definitely feel it, but it isn't overwhelming because the rest of your body isn't in the water.

A few weeks later, Tiffany returned to my office with a twinkle in her eye.

"Aundi, I almost can't believe it. I did it. I mean, you were right, she didn't react well, but I was able to say what I needed to say, and in the end, I'm grateful I did it because even though she doesn't understand my boundaries, she committed to respecting them."

Reader, as you consider your own experience, I invite you to ask yourself these questions to be empowered and prepared in difficulty:

1. Do I have an upcoming situation or experience for which I feel gaining more support would be helpful?

   My situation is: _____

   _____.

2. As you are able, ask yourself, *What do I notice in my body when I think about doing* _____?

It may be helpful to tap into our somatic vocabulary (see page 147) as you consider this question. Feel free to write as little or as much as needed here; your main goal is simply to bring awareness to the needs your body might have. If at any point this exercise feels too overwhelming, please know you may stop and practice grounding, containment, or any other resource you need.

Finally, it's important to recognize that if something is truly too overwhelming, you may wish to revisit it with the help of a therapist or another supportive person at a different time. As I often say, there is no shame in honoring the pace of your body.

And if one topic feels too overwhelming, you may choose to restart the exercise with a topic that feels more tolerable. It will still help you build your emotional flexibility and expand your window of tolerance, which is the ultimate goal.

3. If it feels like it would be supportive, create a future video that will allow you to visualize doing your hard thing.[28]

   a. First, ask yourself: *What would success look like in this experience?* (Focus on what you can control.) Examples might include: staying calm when your child is having a tough time, speaking up in a meeting with colleagues and believing it's brave to do so, following through on setting a boundary, or completing a challenging task without shaming yourself.

   b. Next, consider this question: *What resources do I need to navigate this situation in alignment with my goals and values?* (As a reminder, a resource is anything that helps communicate safety to your body.) Feel free to get creative with this practice and utilize anything I've already named in the book or anything you have experienced in your life as a resource.

   c. Visualize the upcoming event you identified as though it were a video in your mind (i.e., envision yourself arriving where you're going and procedurally going through the event). However, as you do, see if you can also "bring" the resources you named with you, similar to the way Tiffany did. For example, you may wish to visualize yourself actually taking a deep breath before you engage your hard thing. Or you may visualize yourself saying supportive statements to yourself throughout the video.

   d. Once you have a general idea of what your video will be, and it feels like you have enough resources to stay in your window of tolerance while visualizing it, try to run it through at least three times. Additionally, if you are certain this video feels supportive and doesn't feel overwhelming to your system, you may wish to add in tapping each time you run the video. (For a reminder on tapping, check out the resources at the end of chapter 6.)

Remember, this video is now a resource you can return to as often as you need as you prepare for an upcoming challenge.

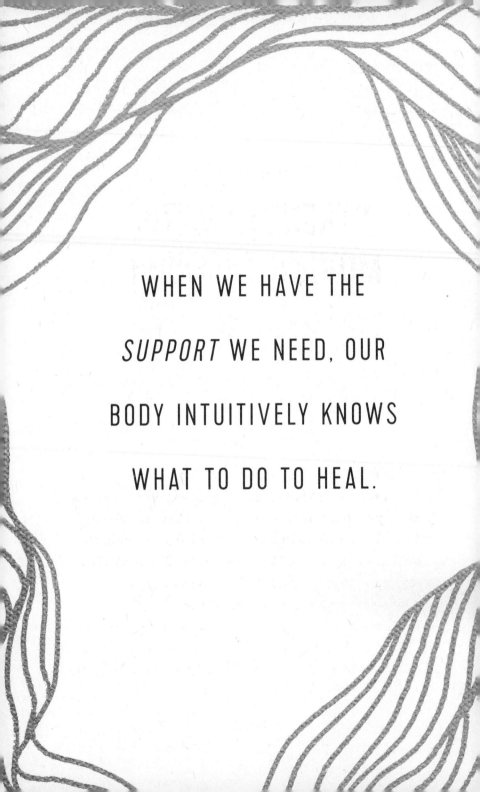

WHEN WE HAVE THE
SUPPORT WE NEED, OUR
BODY INTUITIVELY KNOWS
WHAT TO DO TO HEAL.

CHAPTER 8

STRENGTH WITH MOVING THROUGH

There is no place so awake and alive as the edge of becoming.

SUE MONK KIDD

IN MARCH 2020, I watched, anxious and stunned, as country by country, state by state, the world shut down, unequivocally altered by the reality of COVID-19. It was like I was viewing the world through two lenses: one as a trauma therapist; the second as a person who, like everyone else, had never been through a pandemic before. Trying to process world events through either lens felt surreal and overwhelming.

As the first weeks passed, my family and I began to feel profound exhaustion almost all the time. It was as if we were constantly walking through sludge. With my therapist hat on, this makes sense: Like so many others, we were trying to juggle remote learning for our second-grade daughter, wrangle our active three-year-old son, and transition the very in-person work that Brendan and I do to remote formats. We were grateful to be able to stay home, as so many frontline workers didn't have that option. And yet, the fact remained: We were far beyond a normal kind of tired.

It was a curious experience—carrying the weight of the collective anxiety, uncertainty, fear—as well as our own concerns. But in some ways, this visceral experience was not totally unfamiliar to me. I had often lived with this type of heaviness—the kind that can suck all the energy out of a room. A month or so into the pandemic, I reflected to my husband, "Oh, I think I know why this feels familiar to me. I felt this a lot as a kid—the weight of the world." When there was nowhere to put all the pain, anxiety, and hurt, I just carried it around with me like a huge wet blanket.

Interestingly, I began hearing this same theme of heaviness from many of my clients: Though this was everyone's first pandemic, it was not the first time they'd lived with this kind of exhaustion and frozenness. In fact, seeing much of the world get a small taste of what they'd lived with for decades helped normalize some of my clients' experience with trauma. Each news cycle seemed to report on surging numbers of cases somewhere, even as experts publicly disagreed over how the virus was transmitted. In some small ways, the unpredictability and volatility helped my clients understand why their bodies had responded to disturbing and overwhelming experiences by going into various states of hyper- and hypoarousal. Gratefully, I was able to identify this feeling in my own life fairly early on in the pandemic. My body had often moved into various states of hypoarousal while growing up in order to protect me when there was no escaping my circumstances. Once I honored this young part of me, I began to attune my own compassionate resourcing for what my nervous system was experiencing that spring.

Our bodies are made to move *through* experiences, if we're able.[1] I wondered and prayed often for wisdom to know how I could resource my kiddos in this time. How could I support them so that this collective pain wouldn't become trauma and stay stuck in their little bodies?[2]

On one particular day, the mood in our house felt like a pressure cooker—everyone ready to lash out at any given moment. Tia and Jude had been working hard to be kind to each other, but after weeks of shutdowns, canceled trips, and snowstorms, they were feeling the angst.

"Mooommm!!" they yelled in unison as yet another argument broke out. After we were able to help them take a deep breath following what felt like their hundredth argument of the day, Brendan and I tried something new.

I placed a beanbag chair in the middle of the living room and cranked up some spunky kids' pop music. And then, magic: Tia and Jude began to run and skip in circles around the beanbag. A look of glee and celebration filled their faces as they moved their bodies freely. Brendan and I plopped on the couch with our hands up, ready to give a high-five as they completed each lap around the room. After three or four songs—and a dance party to boot—we were all breathless and sweaty.

As we wound down for bedtime, I could tell that each of us felt a bit more like ourselves.

It didn't change our circumstances; we weren't suddenly happy to be in a pandemic or glad there was so much that was hard in the world. But though it was no magic solution, on many nights we enacted this sort of end-of-day ritual, knowing each of us needed ways to move the stress through our bodies. At least we felt more confident that we would find a way through.

MOVING THROUGH THE STRESS CYCLE

Certainly, running around a beanbag chair didn't and wouldn't solve all our problems. But even this small ritual began to matter to our family. We had created a space, almost a bubble of safety, where Tia and Jude could let their bodies move through the stress and intensity they were undoubtedly feeling.

Because their prefrontal cortexes aren't completely developed, children lack the physiological capacity to regulate themselves or independently process intense sensations, emotions, and experiences.[3] They need the support of a regulated adult with whom they can co-regulate and so move through the swells that come. This movement "through the waves" is more than an idea or theoretical experience. In fact, it's a neurobiological reality: Once we know we're safe, our bodies can metabolize the excess energy that accrues when stress or threat is present.[4]

Children who receive good-enough support and care begin to learn to intuitively ask the questions: *What do I need? Who could help me? What might that look like? How could I move?*[5]

Moving through the waves to find safety? It works for adults too.

Therapist Peter Levine, founder of Somatic Experiencing (a type of body-centered therapy) and author of *Waking the Tiger*, posits that our body is naturally designed to "discharge . . . energy by fleeing or defending itself." When this happens, it will "resolve the threat, [and] trauma will not occur."[6] Though our family wasn't dealing with a threat like being chased by a tiger, our nervous systems were validly detecting the threats brought on by the pandemic.[7] As we've discussed in previous chapters, if our bodies detect threat, their protective mechanisms ramp up. We needed to metabolize all the energy borne from these mechanisms, lest it be stored as trauma.

For Tia and Jude, running around the beanbag helped them "discharge" the excess energy in their bodies brought on by stress. It supported them in two ways: by enabling them to release that stress and *also* by providing cues of safety[8] and goodness in relation to that experience. Instead of locking the sensations of anxiety and fear into their bodies (thus activating only situational strength), they will likely also remember what it felt like to giggle as they released the stress through movement. Brendan and I had helped our kids complete a stress cycle.[9]

However, what happens when we don't have any place to use all of that survival energy? If such stress isn't metabolized or brought to completion[10]—it can get stuck in our bodies and potentially turn into trauma.[11] We try to bury it or avoid it, but it comes out sideways; instead our bodies are dysregulated and act out of situational strength. It comes out in irritation, anxiety, anger, and the confusing sadness whose source you can't quite put your finger on. Sometimes it may even come out in chronic pain or chronic illness.[12]

Allowing a stress cycle to play out, on the other hand, is a little like taking a windup toy, twisting the knob, and then giving it the space it needs to unwind. We have to make room so that all the energy doesn't remain inside, unused.

Amazingly, when we have the *support* we need, our body intuitively knows what to do to heal.[13] It is endowed with a God-given propensity to metabolize and complete physiological cycles. The apostle Paul seems to point to our innate sense to seek redemption and transformation as well: "We know that all creation has been groaning as in the pains of childbirth . . . for we long for our bodies to be released from sin and suffering" (Romans 8:22-23, NLT).

As we work to become more resilient and resourceful, may we learn to move stress through our bodies. Ideally, *all* our experiences (even difficult ones) will be fully processed in this way. When they are, several things occur:

1. **The completion communicates to our body that the situation has ended.**[14] How does this happen? After

a disturbing experience, we can intentionally begin to look for cues of safety that will help us return to our window of tolerance. Once we have the where-withal (typically a sign of transitional strength) to connect to a compassionate resource, our body intui-tively returns at least partially to our window, and in doing this, the systems of our body that are designed to metabolize difficulty are enacted and fully "digest" the experience, sensation, or emotion.[15] In the previ-ous example with our children, Brendan's and my support of Tia and Jude provided the compassionate resource that facilitated our kids "moving through."

2. **The experience can now be stored in our long-term memory** rather than in the right hemisphere of our amygdala (a part of the survival brain, where it is more apt to be activated through the lens of trauma). This is key because, now that the experience has been saved correctly, the neural network is *open* to reflection, learning, and support.[16]

3. **We intuitively begin to make meaning of the expe-rience** rooted in the most accurate version of real-ity.[17] Once we move an experience through our body, we more precisely assess what is actually happening because we are back in our WOT, rather than project-ing from past experiences, which influence how we experience the present. This is a prime signal that an

event is moving through or has already fully metabolized and the cycle has been completed. We can reflect on the experience while remaining regulated and move toward supportive resources going forward.

In many ways, this is where our most expansive strength is truly born. Now our brain is functioning in its most adaptive, resilient state. In many ways, this whole process makes me think of what it would be like to be trapped in a snow globe. Every time we have a stress response—such as going into fight or flight—it's like the snow globe is being shaken so we can't see very far in front of us. However, as we move the energy through our body, it's like being in a snow globe as the flakes fall to the bottom. The more the particles settle, the more clarity we have about who we are, what we need, and what actually happened. (For example, after a difficult experience at work, you may internally reflect on the event like this: *Yes, it was extremely difficult that my supervisor treated me that way. That wasn't okay. And I am so proud of myself for advocating for myself and speaking up.*)

Now, of course, life is life, and not every experience is fully processed in our bodies—particularly those that are too overwhelming for our nervous system to metabolize at the time they occur. This can often be true for those of us who experienced significant toxic stress or trauma in childhood,[18] but it's also true for anyone who doesn't have the capacity or safety to process something at any given time. Many people ask me: If I didn't receive the kind of support needed to complete these cycles when they first occurred or if I perhaps never had the security to let my body move through the intensity it needed to, is healing possible?

My dear reader, it absolutely is.

But moving a fragmented memory/experience/sensation toward completion will require more intentionality (meaning, healthy processing won't necessarily happen intuitively). Because of these fragmented experiences, our neuroception is likely keeping us hypervigilant and attuned to threat, stuck in patterns of situational strength. We can be immensely grateful for the wisdom in our bodies—the wisdom that helped us survive disturbing events and cope in their aftermath. Now we can also be grateful for the wisdom that moves us toward healing.

In addition, we must recognize that, as much as ever, it is vital to honor the pace of our bodies in our healing journey. While reprocessing our stories and completing the body's unfinished cycles may be the ultimate goal, it should never be a bigger priority than our well-being. As Robert Frost once wrote, "The best way out is always through."[19] Indeed, this is true, but if I could add an asterisk to Frost's words, I would say this: While the best way out may *ultimately* be through, it's essential to do that in a way and at a pace that doesn't cause more harm. Ideally, the honoring of pacing will be generative and will create more flexibility in our nervous system—this in turn will allow our full selves to flow toward healing.

One of the most life-giving aspects of my work is helping clients understand that they can offer that support to themselves *now*.

EVERY CYCLE LOOKS FOR COMPLETION

"Aundi, I am so proud of myself!" Luisa leaned forward in her chair, smiling broadly, at the start of our session. "Remember that neighbor I told you about—the one I really like but who at times can be super pushy? I know she means well, but she sometimes makes me feel overwhelmed. I want to know my neighbors and be able to connect, but every time I say no, it feels like she won't accept it or she'll try to pressure me into committing to stuff I'm not comfortable with. Anyway, it happened again . . . but this time, I was finally able to set some kind but firm boundaries. I actually told her directly, 'Hey, I really appreciate you inviting me, but if I say no, I need you to respect that.'"

Luisa took a deep breath, but I could see her still thinking about the encounter. "Well, there is one more thing. Something about all of this still feels unfinished," Luisa continued. "I'm glad I did what I did and I truly do feel proud of myself. But I still have this anxious energy like I'm going to get in trouble or something."

"Could you tell me a little more about what you mean, Luisa?" I asked her.

"Well, I know I did the right thing. And she told me she doesn't completely get where I'm coming from, but she'll respect what I asked of her." Luisa paused. "I guess what I'm wondering is, shouldn't it be over now? Why do I *still* feel anxious and scared?"

"Hmm. I see what you mean, Luisa," I replied. "And I'm proud of you too. What you did isn't easy. I wonder, do you remember that we talked about how important it is to let stress move through your body? So let's say you feel anxious because you were almost hit by a car as you were crossing the street a few minutes ago. That anxiety doesn't necessarily just dissipate. Instead, we have to let our bodies metabolize—or what you and I usually call *move through* the sensation—in order for it to fully process.

"I'd like to support you as you get curious about what you might need to do to allow this experience with your neighbor to fully move through your body. First, though, could I ask you a couple of quick questions?"

"Oh sure, sure," Luisa said as her leg wiggled, cuing me to the anxiety she was feeling.

I led Luisa through a grounding exercise first—just to ensure that she felt some connection to her window of tolerance. At that point, Luisa told me she still felt the anxiety, but from a bit more distance.

Next I led her through a series of questions. "Luisa, where in your body are you noticing this anxiety?" I prompted.

Luisa took several moments to consider my question, and finally she answered, "I just keep feeling this knot in my stomach that I think is a combination of panic and dread. And maybe a sensation like my throat might close up."

Luisa's voice was muted and her lip quivered a little—but I saw determination in her eyes.

"Okay, Luisa. Do you still feel connected to your window as you tell me this?" I asked her gently.

"Yes, yes I do. But it's definitely not comfortable."

"Okay, I want you to remember I'm right here with you. If at any point you want to stop what we're doing, please just let me know. I also want to invite you to place a hand on your stomach and/or your throat as you're noticing that discomfort."

Luisa did so, and I could see her exhale as she felt her own support.

I continued, "Luisa, you're doing a great job. And now, I want you to check in with yourself and see if any of these sensations you're experiencing feel connected to any other experiences?"

Luisa took a moment and was able to identify that this experience made her feel young—perhaps five or six. She was about that age when her family moved in with her grandparents for several years because money was extremely tight. And though she loved her grandpa, he held an incredibly authoritarian view of raising children. He would often yell at Luisa, especially when both her parents were at work. Luisa told me that she felt so overwhelmed she would often tremble and become speechless. Later though, Luisa learned just to fall in line and watch for signs that her grandpa was getting angry.

This new living arrangement also meant that Luisa suddenly lost much of the freedom she'd once enjoyed. Before, in her parents' home, she'd felt free to speak up at dinner, express herself through her clothing choices, ask questions about her faith, or even just laugh loudly. But once they'd moved in with her grandparents, Luisa felt like she was constantly waiting to get in trouble or be cut down.

"I hadn't thought about that with my grandpa in a long time. But this neighbor of mine—she brings me right back to that young little girl who's constantly afraid of getting yelled at, just for being herself," she finished.

Using her situational strength, Luisa learned to walk on eggshells—first around her grandpa, but later around anyone whom her body perceived was similar to him in any way. A younger part of herself was still stuck in situational strength and needed compassionate resourcing to support her in moving forward. Though there are many ways we can move through a cycle when an experience brings up intense emotion (or contain it, if needed), for Luisa, our work tapped into her need to set some embodied boundaries in the present. In a practical sense, Luisa's actions now were on behalf of a younger part of herself who felt trapped and still felt she had to fawn over (appease) her grandpa. Though she had spoken up with her neighbor, it was as though the anxiety in her chest was her younger self asking her to help in that way too.

In the session, we tried a few things that would give Luisa the compassionate resourcing she needed. First, I asked her to notice the sensation of anxiety coursing through her chest. Once she did, I encouraged her to push firmly against a wall in my therapy room while picturing her current self letting her grandpa know she wasn't okay being treated that way.

Luisa was doing this on behalf of her younger self, and the physical act of pushing against the wall was giving sensory input to her body that helped her experience a sense of pushing away her grandpa's power over her, a literal boundary she wasn't able to set when she was young.

"Luisa, you're doing such a good job. I'm wondering if you could check in with yourself again. Do you need another resource here so it feels finished? What does your body want to do right now?"

Luisa's eyes were shiny with tears, and her voice cracked, but she knew right away: "I want to walk away from my grandpa. I want to grab the hand of my younger self and walk away because I said what I needed to say, and we don't need to stay there anymore."

So that's what we did.

As I led her through a visualization in which she escorted her inner child to safety and peace, Luisa was able to move through the cycle of stress that had gotten stuck in her body. She had successfully and compassionately resourced the part of her story that was still stuck in situational strength. This moment was vital to her unlearning the pattern she had developed so long ago. This moment enabled her to experience a new level of repair.

MOVING THROUGH WITH REPATTERNING

To help our bodies discover better ways to respond to difficult circumstances, we often have to release any locked-up traumatic energy from the past or present and learn to *repattern* our body's response during situational strength. This allows us to flow into transitional strength; our body perceives that it is now safe to try something new.

Repatterning not only helps us process past pain or trauma,[20] it also helps us lay new neural pathways to support us in a different physical response. Although it's important to attend to how trauma is stored in the brain, therapist and author Dr. Arielle Schwartz notes that "it is equally important to attend to the impact of trauma on the body."[21] As we learn to establish safety and the ability to maintain dual awareness, our nervous system begins to match its response to our current experience.

For example, as she was growing up, Allie was constantly shamed by her parents and peppered with questions about every significant choice she made. As an adult, whenever a doctor or anyone else she perceived to be an authority asked her a fairly neutral question, she could feel her body automatically brace and her situational strength become activated, which often kept her disconnected from any support that might be available to her. Based on decades of experience with her parents, Allie's nervous system had come to expect any such questions to have a searing impact on her. Yet as Allie has worked to honor her story, compassionately resource her relational trauma, and repattern her body's automatic response to supportive or neutral questions, she has come to learn that, by listening to what her body needs in these situations, she can stay open and curious. From an integrated brain and body, she has more choices about how to act.

This is what happened for Luisa too. As her body was able to move through the cycle and repattern the response she'd developed with her grandpa, she felt free to live differently—to be her full self with her neighbor rather than fawning to meet her every need at any cost.

A major need for focused repatterning in my own life has been my response to incoming electronic messages, such as emails, texts, and voice mails. Several years ago, someone I loved began sending me abusive messages via these channels, and for quite some time afterward I experienced significant body memories (flashbacks that I could *feel* viscerally in my body) when I received any message—even if it wasn't from that person, even if it was completely neutral. I did a lot of processing of the original trauma, and then I began to compassionately resource myself to complete the cycle of trauma that lingered in my body. Becoming aware of my body helped me realize when I needed to soften my jaw, support the knot in my stomach, address the strain in my neck, and slow my heart rate because I'd received a message that felt activating.

I'll be honest: There are still times I notice these patterns in my body (especially if I'm fatigued or worn out). The difference is that I now have the resources to honor and move through whatever arises. Those of us whose bodies carry the heavy imprints of trauma are doing the brave work of becoming strong like water every time we bring safety and support to what our bodies are experiencing. We can learn to repattern our trauma responses so that instead of merely helping us survive, they act *in service of our wholeness and integrated strength.*

LOVE OF NEIGHBOR MOVES US THROUGH

These days, so much information comes our way via news, social media, and other types of communication that simply knowing what's happening in the world can be a little (or a lot) overwhelming. As a trauma survivor myself, I have had to learn how to both honor the bigness of my heart and to care for others, while also figuring out what it means to honor my own limits and needs. It's not easy work.

And yet I find much elegance and beauty in Jesus' simple commandment to "Love your neighbor as yourself" (Mark 12:31). First—and I think this matters a great deal—Jesus' inclusion of "as yourself" reveals what neuroscience has since come to show us: Our bodies are literally unable to attune to the experiences of others if we are disconnected from ourselves.[22]

Not only does Jesus' command remind us that we must love ourselves and that loving our neighbors matters to the well-being of all people, it can also motivate us to mobilize and move through a stress cycle when we've experienced disturbing, overwhelming, or potentially traumatizing events. How does this occur? Though much healing work happens when we turn inward, it is *also* true that healing happens when, as we are able, we turn outward—toward our neighbors who need support.

Prompts to Consider as You Think about Repatterning[23]

1. Briefly scan your body from head to toe.

2. As you do, take note of what you are experiencing right now. If any part of your body feels "tight or contracted," as Dr. Schwartz describes it, you may benefit from answering the following prompts:

   • Where in your body are you experiencing these sensations (e.g., tension in your neck, trembling hands, pounding heart, heaviness in your chest)? If you notice any of these reactions—or something altogether different—see if you can utilize curiosity to try a different way to move your body:

     For tightness in your shoulders, explore movement or touch.

     For a lump in the throat, explore making different sounds.

Part of what I love about Jesus' words is that there is an implied flow within this concept. It's not love your neighbor *or* love yourself. It's love your neighbor *as* yourself. In so many ways this speaks to the mutuality in which our God exists and which we, as image bearers, share in. After all, the fact that the Trinity is composed of three persons (Father, Son, and Holy Spirit) tells us that we are innately designed for relationship, internally and externally.

That is why we may experience a sense of despair when we see people around us being harmed. It affects us—of course it does. Like all emotion, despair is more than a frame of mind; it is typically associated with moving out of our window of tolerance and going down into hypoarousal (dorsal vagal response). As we've discussed, when this kind of survival energy is activated in our body without being metabolized, it has the potential to become trauma. Sometimes the way we move through is by remaining tethered to our sense of self even as we act on behalf of others. Our Creator gives us a framework for flourishing in these simple words: Love your neighbor *as* yourself.

This framework, in the end, actually accelerates our growth. In his landmark book *The Body Keeps the Score*, Dr. Bessel van der Kolk explains that when people who've experienced upsetting events that could lead to post-traumatic stress or other trauma mobilize their energy to help respond to the disaster, they are less likely to develop full PTSD.[24] Psychologist Peter Levine describes a situation in which someone who was held hostage ultimately helped dig his way out of the confinement. Levine noted that this teen was less impacted by the trauma afterward than he would have been if he had given up or not participated in his escape.[25] Moving toward those who are experiencing pain or working to alleviate suffering can help the people we're assisting, and it may also be good for us.

Of course, here's an important reminder for those of us prone to over-accommodating, people-pleasing, and/or fawning: It's essential that we continue to pay compassionate attention to our

For trembling hands. notice what it feels like to tighten and then loosen them.

For a pounding heart. place your hand on your heart and notice what it feels like to be supported.

For heaviness in your chest. give yourself a bear hug and notice what that support feels like.

Each of the prompts above is merely a suggestion and an invitation to bring curiosity to the way your body may need to move in order to move through the cycle of whatever you're feeling. Please add to or tweak these suggestions based on what you are experiencing.

own experience. In helping others, we must do what we can to stay connected to our window of tolerance. Otherwise, we may lose sight of our own limits and fall back into the protective pattern of fawning, which will ultimately keep us stuck.

However, as we are able, if we can truly listen and love our neighbor as ourselves for love's sake, then we have the opportunity for beauty to unfold. Here we come to truly see that we do, just as Mother Teresa once said, "belong to each other."

BECOMING STRONG LIKE WATER

Throughout this chapter, we've discussed multiple ways that our bodies can and (at the pace we are able) need to move through our experiences. Depending on your own history around trauma, attachment, and mental health, your specific needs for moving through a cycle may vary. This is normal, and a trauma-informed perspective on this work requires that we each attune to the specificities of our own nervous system.

With that said, following are several prompts to help guide you into self-awareness as you work to compassionately resource and mobilize your body to move through painful experiences that have gotten stuck in your body.

TEMPLATES TO COMPASSIONATELY
UNWIND/MOVE THROUGH THE CYCLE

Earlier in this chapter, I showed you how Luisa was able to move through a cycle that had been stuck in her body since childhood, allowing her to bravely face her need to walk on eggshells around others because of her fear of upsetting them. Now I invite you to practice completing some somatic resonance in areas that you cannot seem to move past.

I encourage you to start by connecting with a situation that is only mildly challenging as a way to build up and expand your window:

1. Take a moment to consider a situation, emotion, or sensation that feels stuck. For example, you might notice mild anxiety after watching a television show, dread at the thought of returning work emails, or perhaps a sense of overwhelm about the need to clean your kitchen.

2. Now, from a grounded place, notice what you are experiencing in your body as you think about this situation/emotion/sensation. If it feels supportive, place a hand on your heart or some other part of your body.

3. Next, see if you can use curiosity to ask yourself what is needed for your body to complete the cycle. For example, movement such as swaying, shaking, walking, or even jumping may help you move anxiety through your body. Maybe you wish to turn on a loud, upbeat song and sing along. Perhaps you could experiment with singing, humming, or other sounds such as "voo" (like an ocean liner in fog).[26] Or if you are feeling dread (which is typically connected to a dorsal vagal response), you may need to attentively support this emotion through self-compassion or other resources. If you feel powerless or overwhelmed, this may be a time to take small, resourced steps toward movement or complete a simple task. Alternately, it may be a time to consider a small step toward supporting or helping someone else.

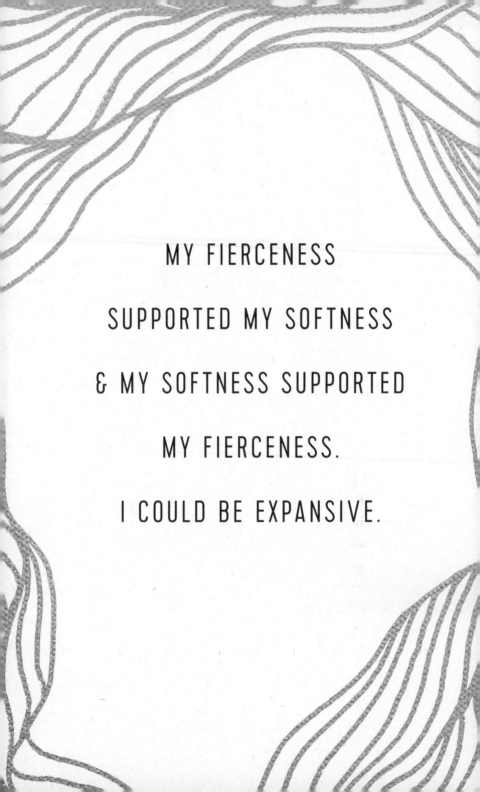

MY FIERCENESS

SUPPORTED MY SOFTNESS

& MY SOFTNESS SUPPORTED

MY FIERCENESS.

I COULD BE EXPANSIVE.

CHAPTER 9

STRENGTH WITH INTEGRATION

It takes courage to grow up and become who you really are.

E. E. CUMMINGS

IN FEBRUARY 2019, our little family traveled to my hometown in the Pacific Northwest, where I would be inducted into my high school's hall of fame as the all-time leading scorer for basketball. Much of my extended family—my mom, siblings, and in-laws—would be there to celebrate with me. Despite everyone's excitement, I felt wobbly and tired, as I had come in just under the wire to complete the manuscript for my first book. That had taken just about every ounce of anything I had to offer.

When we arrived at our rental house, which by design

203

offered a partial view of the ocean, I could feel my shoulders loosen. I watched the waves lap far off in the distance. I smelled the salty air and took in the clouds, which were, as usual, gray and broody. In that moment, I had a sense of the sacredness of this time; of what a privilege it was for me to return to places where I had experienced so much pain and also so much joy. It felt almost serendipitous, like God had set a table for me right there; a special kind of homecoming. I was grateful to experience the Spirit's nearness as I knew this weekend would bring up many different emotions.

For many years, especially early in my recovery from childhood trauma, I struggled to know what to do with the fierce, powerful part of myself that showed up on the basketball court. I felt at odds with my own strength, which I see now was often situational. And so in response, I felt that I needed to shame or disconnect from this element of myself. That self—the one full of determined grit and intensity—scared me. I loved her, but at times I was almost afraid of her; maybe even angry with her that she hadn't helped me in other areas of my life when I needed it.

In many ways—especially in a culture that often doesn't affirm strength in women—I assumed I had to choose between being a certain kind of strong or a certain kind of gentle. My picture of healing was sometimes narrow; I didn't yet recognize that I didn't have to choose between my fierceness or my softness. They were both me. In fact, as the ancient Chinese philosopher Lao Tzu once wrote, "What is soft is strong." I was also inspired by psychologist Kristin Neff to recognize that my fierceness supported my softness and my softness supported my fierceness.[1] I could be expansive. Not when I cut off parts of myself, but when I allowed their full, God-given expression.

It was time to truly be with and honor this younger part of myself, the one who had shown up in the world in the best way she knew how. Her situational strength was formidable. I finally felt safe enough to allow this younger version of me, along with all she had experienced, to be integrated into my full self.

What do I mean when I talk about integration? Through compassionate resourcing, I had learned to move along the flow of strength. No longer did I feel as if I needed my situational strength only to stay alive; instead, my strength could work in service of my integration—my wholeness. This *integrated strength* meant that my body was fully rooted in my true self, firmly planted in my WOT. From this strength, I knew in my very bones that we are made to live *from* Love and not for it.

Importantly, I had also realized that even when something did activate my situational strength—whether past wounds or truly threatening circumstances in the present—my body had learned how to surf the waves that came my way until I could move through what I was experiencing and return to integrated strength.

Once I'd accepted the invitation to return to my high school and had prepared to see many people from my past and discuss my years on the court, I realized that I felt supported, loved, and resourced, both externally *and* internally. What a difference it made to my younger self that I didn't feel as if the world rested on her shoulders anymore.

You May Be in Integrative Strength When You Experience:

- Presence: *I feel truly in this moment.*
- Completeness: *Whew, it's over now.*
- Clarity: *Oh, I think I can see the bigger picture.*
- Openness: *Maybe I could try something new.*
- Feeling Capable: *I know I can do this because I've done this before.*
- Authenticity: *It's okay to be who I truly am.*
- Feeling Empowered: *I have the support and resources I need to do this thing.*
- Hope: *There are so many possibilities of what could happen next.*
- Feeling Safely Embodied:[2] *It feels good to be in my body.*
- Pro-Social: *There are people who are really for me. It not only feels safe to connect with the people I care about, it feels good.*

As I sat around tables with old friends and former coaches, took walks along the beach, and celebrated this prestigious award, I felt a deepened gratitude toward my fierce younger self. I felt connected with her in a way I'd never experienced before. In my younger years, the intensity I felt when connected to my situational strength was so big that at times I was sent out of my limited window of tolerance. But now, after working to honor my story, build safety, expand my window, and draw on compassionate resources, it felt as though this younger part of myself finally believed that I was an adult.

I didn't need to become less of myself but more. God wasn't asking me to get rid of this beautiful part of myself. Instead, I could honor all parts of me so they could come into alignment with whom He had made me to be.

The second-century church leader Irenaeus is believed to have written, "The glory of God is the human person fully alive." What a powerful reminder that just as Jesus became a man and lived an incarnational life, we are ultimately invited to live that way too. After all, we are made in the image of our incarnational, alive God. That is what I want: to be fully and deeply alive. And yet for so many (valid) reasons, we may experience a disconnect from this experience. What hope for each of us as we move along the flow of strength, to know that it is "from his fullness [that] we have all received, grace upon grace" (John 1:16, ESV).

During that weekend, I realized something new about the work of becoming strong like water: My truest, most profound strength will never be found in denying the reality of my personhood or my story. Instead, the deepest strength has always, always been about welcoming them home.

THE RETURN IS PART OF INTEGRATION

One blessing I've prayed over both myself and others a lot during the last few years is this: "May you be met in the fullness of your humanity." I understand this can be complicated for many people. And to be fair, it is challenging. It is not easy to be human these days. We are both so beloved and yet so very fragile. In our vulnerability, it's tempting to want to keep certain parts hidden. We want to outthink our trauma. We want to "outlogic" our pain. We want to run, to protect, to suppress, to pretend. I get it. And as we've discussed, sometimes our bodies simply do the best they can to help us navigate the hard.

Consider my client Denise. She had a history of complex trauma from childhood abuse but had worked for years to recognize and heal from its effects. One day as she sat down in my office at the start of our session, she let out a deep sigh. "I feel so frazzled," she said. "I promised myself that I wouldn't overextend myself by volunteering at my kids' school on top of starting my new role as a manager—but this past month I kept breaking my word to myself. Then, I found myself yelling at my kids, even though I'm the one I'm angry at. Ugh. After healing for this long, I just feel like that shouldn't happen anymore, you know?"

Like many of my clients, Denise found it discouraging to "think" that she'd completely overcome something—only to find it showing up in her life again. As both a trauma survivor and a therapist, I've found it essential to normalize the idea that sometimes, even after having done a lot of work, we will still leave ourselves. Occasionally we will find ourselves leaving our window of tolerance, even about a situation we thought we'd healed from. We may find ourselves turning back to a coping skill that isn't currently helpful (though perhaps, at some point, it may have helped us survive difficulty). Or we may say yes even when we meant to say no. We may discover that we feel disconnected and fragmented, even though we're doing all the "right" things.

We are not static beings who are planted in one way and place for all time. Instead, we have the God-given capacity to change, grow, and heal; we can return. From a faith lens, we can remember God's movement toward us before we even knew we needed Him. We can think of the verse "We love because he first loved us" (1 John 4:19). God created us with the intention to never leave us.

He also invites us to turn back toward Him. In the Christian tradition, the Greek word *metanoia*, which is often translated "repentance," means to have a change of mind.[3] It's sometimes paired with the Greek word *epistrephō*,[4] which conveys the idea that a person can "turn oneself about" or "turn back."[5] These two words are used to convey the act of repenting from sin or wrongdoing toward God. And there is great value to this. Sometimes we do need to turn away from the harm we are causing and make amends—to others, God, or ourselves. But even when we have been the one wronged, there is value in noticing when we can't continue down a certain path, then turning away from it and turning toward *life*; toward the Life Giver.

In a sense, all integration is a return. Even when we begin to lose our aim, our focus, our integrity, our compassion—maybe even our hope—the truth is that "the healing is in the return,"[6] as mindfulness teacher Sharon Salzberg says. I love God's wisdom in recognizing and embedding this into who we are. *We are made for the return.*

From a trauma lens, we can recognize and honor the fact that unresolved pain and trauma create fragmentation. Sometimes this fragmentation *is* the only way to survive in a particular moment. I don't say that flippantly. I've sat with some folks whose trauma was so severe and overwhelming that simply to be present in their bodies was a profound victory. At times in my own trauma recovery, I've felt as if staying present in my own body required me to carry what felt like the literal weight of the world. I've seen this with my own eyes and felt it in my own being. And yet I also believe that God's tenderness—His

loving-kindness—to us in our pain is beyond human understanding. No wonder visceral psychological safety supports us
in our return to goodness. We don't return out of fear, though
that may be present. We return because we are designed for
connection, fullness, and abundance. We return because God
invites us to be whole; and every time we return to God and
ourselves, our ability to be strong like water grows.

REST IS A PART OF HEALING

Often, particularly after we've faced something difficult,
overcome hardship, processed pain, or simply experienced
something intense (even if good), our bodies need time and
support to rest. The rest allows us to fully process and move
through our experiences. This rhythmic nature is the way
all of creation functions. As Ecclesiastes 3:1 says, "There is
a time for everything, and a season for every activity under
the heavens." We were made to flow like water. We simply
cannot and were not made to be in one season at all times.

There is undoubtedly an ebb and flow to being human,
and that is no accident. Our Creator knows how vital and
foundational rest is to our well-being. It's such an important
concept that God commanded the Jewish people to take a
full day every week to cease labor on the Sabbath.

If you've carried the heavy burdens of trauma, abuse,
neglect, and/or other forms of unprocessed pain, you may
feel as if there has never been rest from this pain; almost like
there has never been a real Sabbath. You may have adapted

to this pain by developing intense situational strength; but reader, you don't have to keep carrying this weight. As you are able, you are invited to set it down. I suppose this is what keeps me so tethered to Jesus. When the God of the universe says, "Come to me, all you who are weary and burdened, and I will give you rest" (Matthew 11:28), every part of my spirit says yes. Partly because that burden, which includes the neuroception (see page 64) and energy required to maintain hypervigilance or some form of disconnection, *is* labor.

A while ago, I jotted a note to myself on the notes app in my phone where I keep so many different ideas. I wrote this: *Deep work requires deep rest.* Often, I come back to this simple line as a way to ground myself in the work that I do. It would be easy to bypass and override how much it matters that we allow our bodies to recover after challenge. After all, this is how much of our culture encourages us to function. But the wisdom of strong like water is different; it reminds us that we are cyclical beings more than linear ones. And that ultimately, rest must be a part of healing.

Keep going but take breaks

By the end of our short Oregon trip, not only had I been inducted into my high school's sports hall of fame, but I'd experienced the profound with-ness of God and felt a deep hospitality toward my younger self. In other words, I had done some serious integrating. I noticed, though, how much I had needed the *space* to let that happen. Miraculously, even with a full schedule, I experienced a spaciousness I couldn't explain.

I waded through thick green brush with my kids, Brendan, my in-laws, my mom, and my siblings. I allowed my body to unwind more deeply than I had for a long time. I just *was*. I simply tried to be present—to smell the salty air that spoke to the center of my soul. We cooked, laughed, and caught up. After several years of intense trauma work in my own life, I felt more whole on these familiar barren and rocky beaches than maybe ever before.

And then as our trip came to a close, the weirdest, most unexpected thing happened: It snowed. On the beach. Which happens exactly never (okay, every once in a while it does happen). It's not uncommon to see a thick blanket of white where we lived in Colorado, but I was caught by delighted surprise when I woke up in our rental house and saw a pink sunrise on the beach surrounded by pine trees covered in snow.

We had to drive all the way back to Portland for our flight, so in the early hours, my mom came over to help us pack. After my kiddos blew her their last kisses, I leaned over to hug my mom and say goodbye. I found myself taking a second look at her. I remembered how brave she has had to be: to heal from her own trauma; to practice sobriety; to leave an abusive marriage; to rebuild her life after so much harm; to do the hard work of reparations with me and others.

"Keep going, Mom," I said as I squeezed her tight. "But take breaks. Okay?"

She exhaled. I watched her shoulders drop. My mom grinned back at me, her eyes shiny with tears, and said,

"Oh honey, you too. With everything: the book, the kids, therapy—all of it. Keep going. But take breaks. I love you."

Many of us intuitively know that the only way to truly work through something is to face it directly. To feel it. To see it. To do it. To live it. Yet, as we know from our work in this book, a classic view of pushing ourselves until we break doesn't actually lead to resilience. There is wisdom in the rhythms of our bodies that helps us to understand when to move forward and when to pause, rest, ask for help, or connect with deeper resources. This is where a more holistic, expansive strength is born.

When we learn to listen to this wisdom, we find that not only can we move through difficulty, but also we may discover a renewed sense of purpose in the world. I see it all the time in my therapy practice:

- The woman who grew up with hypercritical parents finds the courage to disappoint others and finally pursues her vocational passion.
- The man who felt weak for acknowledging his sadness learns to grieve in therapy and then creates a peer-led grief group.
- The sexual abuse survivor who never thought she could advocate for herself finds she has a gift for law.
- The client healing from trauma finds her voice and begins to speak out against injustice.

You see, when someone finally has the safety, resources, and support to fully honor their experiences, not only can they work through their past, but they can also dream about possibilities for their future.

WE'RE NOT PROJECTS

Most nights Brendan and I tag team bedtime for Tia and Jude. One of us may be in the bathroom helping with teeth, while the other is making sure pj's are on and other tiny needs are attended to. Occasionally though, one of us is traveling or working late.

This is what happened one crisp fall night, when I found myself exhausted at bedtime. Actually, strike that—I was utterly fried. I decided to leave the dishes in the sink and let go of several little tasks I had wanted to get done. Part of my own growth in the last decade has been to make sure I'm prioritizing my people and my presence over that which won't matter in the end. Certainly, this has been (and still is) a growth area for me.

But I was glad that I did make space for even the tiniest chance to connect in the midst of a chaotic day because I found myself struck by the question my four-year-old son asked just after we'd read a children's version of the Creation story from Genesis 1. "Mama," Jude asked quietly, "are we projects to God? Like, does God want to make sure we're finished and then move on to something else?"

Jude had just crawled into his bed, and I was beginning to pull up his blanket, but his question stopped me in my tracks. Though it had been quite a long day in the middle of many, many long days, my heart felt like it might burst. I looked over into his inquisitive, chocolate-brown eyes and felt such deep love for this little person who is just beginning to ask big, important questions. In just the past few days he had asked me how engines work, how birds fly, what happens in a tornado, how people feel their emotions, and what I do at work. The whys were endless—but I knew the question he was asking now mattered a whole lot. I also knew we'd likely revisit the answer to this particular one again and again as he grows, especially in a culture that so often commodifies and objectifies the human experience. It felt vital to make sure Jude knew how deeply he is loved by me, his dad, his family, and his Creator—not because there was something to fix, but because we were made as image bearers.

"Oh, love, that's a great question." I cuddled him close. "No, no, we're not projects to God. We're more like his kids. Just like if you were having a hard time, Mommy and Daddy would stay close and do all we could to help you, God is like that with us too. Except God is always with us, in a way even Mommy and Daddy can't be. So, no, baby, we're not projects."

A few minutes later, I sat on our couch by myself and thought about what Jude had asked me. It can be so challenging to keep healing and hoping. Yet we do, because it's never been about a finish line or where we've landed on the flow of strength. Instead, it's always been about the fact that our truest identity is that we are beloved. This, I've come to believe, is what allows us to keep returning, to keep coming home to ourselves again and again.

BECOMING STRONG LIKE WATER
CALLING BACK ALL PARTS OF OURSELVES[7]

A normal part of being human is losing our way at times. Even after we have learned something new or experienced some elements of healing, we may still find ourselves making a wrong turn, harming others or ourselves, failing to act on something we know to be true, or falling back into situational strength and other old patterns that no longer serve us.

In such times, I remember how sweet these words from Scripture are: "The LORD longs to be gracious to you" (Isaiah 30:18). Dear reader, when you find yourself thinking or acting in a way that no longer aligns with who God has made you to be, I hope you can steward generous compassion toward yourself *in that same way.*

In this practice, please ensure you are feeling grounded and present to the space you are in. As always, please be sure you have at least one foot in your window of tolerance in order to honor your body's pace.

Now I invite you to visualize any emotion, pattern, or part of yourself that feels overextended, disconnected, or in some way fragmented from your true self. For example, you might see yourself saying yes when you meant no. Or you may see yourself scrambling to make something perfect, even when you're bone weary. As you do this, what sensations do you notice in your body? Where are they located?

Next, I suggest that you place one hand on your heart and the other on your stomach to communicate support to your body. In your mind's eye, have your true self invite any emotions, sensations, or parts back to the whole. Visualize a magnet pulling these elements of yourself back in with compassion and care. If it feels helpful, you may wish to bring in an affirmation to repeat to yourself to support you in this process. Examples include:

I can stay with myself.
I can be gentle with myself.
I am beloved.
It's okay to be in process.
I am making progress.
I can come back to myself.
I am responsible for only myself.
It's okay for others to be uncomfortable.
I am allowed to take care of myself.

I invite you to stay with this practice for as long as you need.

HONORING THE INTEGRATION

In this chapter, I share a story about feeling integrated with my younger self, as well as noticing that I had learned to fluidly move along the flow of strength. Take a moment, and as you are able, recall if you have experienced a time in your life when you felt you have moved along the flow of strength. Perhaps this happened in a situation like the one I described with wounds from a younger self, or perhaps it could simply be experiencing situational strength and observing that it processed and moved through your body until it felt completed.

As you consider this, pause to notice what you are experiencing in your body. Do you feel a sense of healthy pride or gratitude? Do you notice a softening, a gentleness, or a sense of love? Do you notice a sense of compassion, admiration, or desire to care for an age or part of yourself?

If it feels helpful, I invite you to place a hand on your heart and savor this moment. As you breathe, remember that every time we take the time to observe moments of integration, we are building a foundation for more integration in the future.

IT'S WHEN WE

LEND COMPASSION TO

PLACES & EXPERIENCES

OF GREAT PAIN, AS WE

ARE ABLE, THAT THE MOST

BEAUTY RISES.

CHAPTER 10

STRENGTH WITH REIMAGINING

I remain confident of this:
I will see the goodness of the LORD in the land of the living.

PSALM 27:13

ONE DAY A FEW MONTHS AFTER MY SON, Jude, was born, I found myself beyond frayed. Jude had several allergies we weren't aware of, and I didn't yet know how to adapt what I ate so my breast milk wouldn't trigger his allergies. On a practical note, his distress meant that I wasn't sleeping.

I was keenly aware that I wasn't anything like the mom I thought I'd be. My house was a mess. My daughter, Tia, wore a tie-dyed shirt with a pink tutu and had bits of breakfast all over her face. I carried sweet Jude in my wrap around our little house because that was the only place he'd sleep. No, seriously—*the only place.* I loved my kids fiercely, but I felt the suffocating sense that I couldn't handle this gig.

As I sat on our couch that day, I thought: *I wonder if I could do this differently.*

That question may not seem like that big of a deal. But for me, it was actually the fruit of years of compassionate resourcing and learning to live strong like water. The thought itself was rooted in the recognition that, when something wasn't working, maybe I shouldn't just harm myself, leave myself, shame myself, or go back to any of the ways I survived in the past. Maybe that wasn't the person my kids needed. Maybe it was time to get creative—*to reimagine.* I had to courageously ask myself, *What do I want to pass on to my kiddos?*

To get to that answer, I needed to reimagine what it might look like to take care of myself so I could mother well. I had to release my efforts to become what I imagined a cookie-cutter type of supermom should be. No, it wouldn't work for me to try to do it all. No, I couldn't do it alone. No, I didn't have unlimited capacity. And yes, I would have to become even more comfortable with disappointing others to honor myself, my family, and my integrity.

Brendan and I began to have long conversations about parenting, vocation, and just about everything else that affected our day-to-day lives. We worked together to reprioritize and redefine success.

It was here, in this muddled, bleary-eyed stage of motherhood, that something new was born in me.

PARTICIPATING WITH GOD IN THE WORK

Sometimes living from a place of generativity and creativity means we appear different from what others desire for and of us. For instance, Jesus was not who the Jewish people or even His followers expected. Instead of a warrior, He was a lowly carpenter. Instead of being raised in a palace, He grew up in a dusty little village. Instead of advocating violence, He preached turning the other cheek. Instead of trying to make a name for Himself or leading with might, Jesus said that "the last shall be first." Instead of pushing children away because they were a nuisance, Jesus invited them to come to Him and honored their humanity. Jesus advocated for the marginalized, and His fiercest words were always for those with the most money, power, and influence. Jesus' entire life was rooted in a higher understanding of God's hope for each of us (see Isaiah 55:8-9). He loved people so deeply; He loves *us* so deeply. Many people projected their hopes, desires, and wants on Jesus. And though He was compassionate, He did not waver in His conviction that He'd been called to bring a different kind of Kingdom.

Jesus understood His assignment.

His Kingdom was not what the disciples expected, so I can empathize with their profound grief when Jesus died a violent death on the cross. Here was the God who at times had befuddled them but whom they had still hoped would save them; here was this God dying a human death. How could this be? Even after everything they had learned and experienced *with* Jesus, they were profoundly disappointed.

However, a part of me wonders if the ways the disciples had experienced Jesus stayed with them as a resource. I can't help but wonder if the tiniest sparks of their time with Him remained below their consciousness. I can't help but wonder if they recalled how they felt in His presence or what it was like to feel peace when by His side. Did they recall His laugh? Did they think about their last conversation with Him? Did they think about the bread being broken? Did the embodied memories of with-ness steady their nervous systems even as they grieved—waiting to participate with God in reimagining what would come next: resurrection?

The truth is, the Bible is silent on these particularities of the disciples' experiences. Yet we know that the experiences of our bodies absolutely matter. I can't tell you how many times I've stood on what feels like the edge of a cliff with someone in their healing work. It can seem like the shadows of pain will never cease, that there will never be a time that things are different. How does a God like ours allow grief to create fertile ground for experiencing things like hope, joy, and ultimately newness? Reader, I don't exactly know. I certainly don't have all the answers here, but like so much of this strong-like-water work, I can honor the mystery.

I think often of the story of young Joseph in Genesis 37–50. Because Joseph was clearly their father's favorite child, his brothers were jealous and sold him to slave traders headed to Egypt. Joseph experienced many ups and downs during the years of his captivity, and he endured much harm, pain, and loss. Ultimately, though, Joseph participated with

God to save many people from famine and was elevated to a lofty position in Egypt. When his brothers finally bowed before him and begged for mercy, he replied with humble confidence, "You planned something bad for me, but God produced something good" (Genesis 50:20, CEB).

Though we know Joseph grieved deeply when he finally revealed his identity to his brothers (see Genesis 45:1-2), I wish I could have seen his posture and heard the tone of his voice when he said these specific words. Can you even imagine? I wonder what kind of internal work and healing Joseph had gone through to get to this point. How many tears had he cried? What kind of emotions did he have to feel? With what kinds of thoughts did he have to wrestle? Based on his response to his brothers, I don't think Joseph was bypassing his trauma; rather, he was acting as a compassionate witness to it. Joseph was able to reimagine the effects of his trauma because he'd come to a place of being compassionately resourced by the God of the universe.

There is so much nuance to each of our stories, and I never want to develop a narrative that defends the way anyone—especially a person with a history of complex trauma—has been harmed. And though I will never celebrate the pain of another, every single time something that had been intended for evil is transformed into something good, I celebrate.

This requires us to hold another paradox: When we participate in reimagining, we are experiencing the goodness of the Lord, and every time we move toward reimagining, we have clearer eyes to see it.

REIMAGINING A NEW WORLD

When I first met my client Alex, he seemed to be at the end of his rope. "I don't know if you can help me, but honestly, I'm willing to try just about anything at this point," he told me one day.

Alex had just withdrawn from an educational program where he'd planned to pursue a master's in public health. Just ten months prior, his closest friend had tragically died in a car accident—with Alex in the passenger seat beside him. On that pivotal day, Alex witnessed and experienced more pain in a single minute than he'd ever thought possible. Understandably, the entire experience left deep imprints of trauma.

Alex felt numb for the first few weeks after the accident, but others wondered if he'd even been affected at all. Inwardly, Alex's body used every ounce of situational strength he could muster to make it through a mere hour of the day. His life became increasingly difficult to manage; for instance, every time he had a moment of stillness, he experienced such severe flashbacks that he grew terrified of quiet—worried the images, sensations, and emotions of the accident would come roaring back.

After we worked together for several months to make sure Alex was compassionately resourced, we began to process the experience in earnest. Over several sessions we used eye movement desensitization and reprocessing (EMDR) to do the hard and involved labor of working through the traumatic memories.

Though it was beyond difficult at times, Alex was profoundly grateful when he could report that our processing had decreased the trauma of the accident almost completely. It was a beautiful, hard-won realization. "Thanks, Aundi. I guess I never thought I'd be able to actually heal. I mean, being with my friend in that accident—it, it ruined my life. I always hoped healing was possible, but . . . yeah. Just . . . thanks," Alex told me with tears in his eyes.

And yet this understanding came with a new fear: What would it look like for him to engage his world *now*? Because of his many PTSD symptoms, Alex had left his previous program and turned down several other opportunities around education and work. His situational strength had helped him survive after the accident, but it had also shrunk his world. The thought of that world expanding was as frightening as it was exhilarating.

Then Alex told me he'd been given the opportunity to move across the country for another prestigious master's program. He'd applied on a whim, sharing the journey he'd been on in therapy to make him a better health advocate for others. To process what that could look like, I offered him the compassionate resource of *reimagining* during our session.

"Alex, as you consider this possible move, take a moment to do a body scan. As you do so, what are you noticing?" I asked him.

"Mostly, I'm noticing a sense of openness in my chest. Almost like, there are possibilities for me," Alex shared.

Next I guided Alex through a future video protocol to

help him visualize what resources he would need to reimagine and move toward this future. As we finished the exercise, the room was silent but Alex was beaming—grinning from ear to ear. I felt a tingle go down my spine because Alex was living the work of strong like water: tapping into the hope he already felt as he paired it with the tangible resources that could help him bring it to fruition.

When we consider the common grace and scientific significance of neuroplasticity[1]—the ability of the brain to adapt, rewire, and change—we are invited to stand back in awe and recognize that not only can our bodies survive unthinkable things, we can heal from them. We can also grow *through* them. As I've said many times (but it bears repeating), I will never celebrate someone's pain, but I will embrace the reality that our God is a God of resurrection.

And this is what it means to be strong like water; to be available to the love that is "strong as death" (Song of Songs 8:6). We honor not only the death, but life. We are present to and in the fullness of our human experience. This, too, is grace. This, too, is strength.

THE POTENTIAL FOR SOMETHING NEW TO BE BORN

I believe God imbued each of us with a sense of what wholeness is and could be. And as humans made in the image of our Creator, we groan and long for that.[2] In our imperfect humanity, however, we certainly don't always move toward this wholeness well.

Sometimes we mistake the gifts for the giver. Sometimes we misunderstand our desires, and in the process of looking for wholeness, even harm ourselves through our addictions or the poor ways we treat ourselves. Yet when we reframe these missteps, seeing them not simply as bad things but as our misguided attempts to move toward goodness, we can bring in self-compassion and appreciation for the ways we can heal and the wisdom our bodies carry. Once we understand that God also wants wholeness for us, we recognize that our ability and desire to heal is a good gift from God: "Every good and perfect gift is from above" (James 1:17).

I nearly weep when I consider the goodness of God displayed through our bodies' desire not only to survive but also to heal. Writing this chapter on reimagining feels special to me for a few reasons. For one, much of what I've written about in this book happened in the past, but I am applying the strong-like-water work of reimagining to my own life right now. I'm living this right alongside you, reader.

Second, the pandemic has either broken us down or revealed the cracks that existed in life before COVID-19. That, in turn, means something new is being formed. At the precise moment I'm typing this, we are entering yet another surge of the pandemic—the fourth wave, I think they're calling it. And like so many people around the world, our little family is exhausted and worn. We've been privileged to have access to most of what we need throughout these last few years, but it has still been costly. We've lost family members, grieved the loss of experiences we hoped would happen, experienced mental health challenges, ached over the collective and personal trauma, and more.

Certainly, I've had to learn to reimagine at times before, but this time feels especially painful. Yet maybe it's sacred too. I'm holding on to this: Often the potential for something new is found in the places where we have experienced and honored grief. This is absolutely part of what happened for Alex in the story above, and for so many of my clients, friends, and other survivors. It's when we lend compassion to places and experiences of great pain, as we are able, that the most beauty rises.

There is a mystery and cycle embedded in the ebb and flow of life. For some reason, loss and lament often create fertile ground for tiny shoots of new life. This is the foundation of what it means to reimagine. Poet, author, and activist James Baldwin said, "Not everything that is faced can be changed; but nothing can be changed *until* it is faced."[3] Baldwin is addressing the need for our country to confront the many shadows of our past, certainly including the deep roots of racism. But I also find myself feeling some hope in his words—a precious alchemy occurs when we finally *turn with compassion toward* the painful elements of our personal and communal stories rather than try to simply suppress, shame, spiritually bypass, or slap some toxic positivity on them.

When we can get to what my friend Steve Carter calls "the thing beneath the thing,"[4] we open ourselves to the possibility of creatively, lovingly, and compassionately finding a new way forward with our God-given imagination. This doesn't mean that we forget the significance of the pain or loss, or that we won't need to repair harm we've done in ourselves or others, but it does mean our relationship to the pain and loss can change.

As we work to integrate the fullness of our stories—the good, the hard, and everything in between—we will have clear eyes to see the possibilities before us. This is the cycle of strong like water: being tethered to safety compassionately resources us so we can feel; feeling allows us to complete the physiological cycle; and moving through the cycle allows us to dream a new dream, hope a new hope.

COURAGEOUS HOPE

Once something has been torn down, a certain kind of hope is required to believe we are capable of reimagining it. This is not easy hope. This is courageous hope. Especially if this hope hasn't been modeled for you. Especially if much of your life has required simply surviving.

"Story follows state," master therapist Deb Dana asserts,[5] which means that as our nervous system experiences regulation and safety, our bodies will intuitively have the capacity to imagine a new story. Reimagining, you see, is not and cannot be produced by our survival brain. Yes, we can honor and be grateful for the way it's helped us, but it is neither creative nor generative. Ultimately, our situational strength is simply and only protective. Only love can truly lead us home; only love can envision something different from the patterns that have kept us stuck.

This is why the work of artists, poets, prophets, writers, and musicians matters so much. Their creativity is the interface of the work of God whispering to us, His beloved, "See, I am doing a new thing!" (Isaiah 43:19). Reimagining is the work of those dedicated to realizing the prophets' call to "let justice roll down like waters, and righteousness like an ever-flowing stream" (Amos 5:24, ESV). I have long loved these words from Dr. Martin Luther King: "I have decided to stick with love. Hate is too great a burden to bear."[6] It's easy to take his statement out of context and assume he's referring to a shallow, false-pretense kind of love—one that wants people to act happy when they're in despair, or to act as though there is peace when there is chaos. But I don't believe that is what he is getting at. Similarly, author, pastor, and anti-racism peacemaker Osheta Moore discusses what seems to be the true foundation of this costly love in her book *Dear White Peacemakers*:

> The whole of Jesus' ministry was to establish a community so convinced of their Belovedness to God that they proclaim the Belovedness of others. Belovedness is a massive act of owning and accepting your humanness as a gift from a God who deeply loves you. As we adjust our thinking of this work as rehumanizing those who have been dehumanized, Belovedness is essential in our anti-racism peacemaking.[7]

I'm grateful for Moore's words; in a world in which we are often celebrated for buckling down and continuing to stay in

survival mode, to pretend, or even to turn toward violence—
the invitation to a sacred reimagining remains.

REIMAGINING BY WAY OF AN OPEN HEART

A few years ago a pastor friend of mine sent me an email
that said something like this: "Aundi, I don't know what it's
cost you to know what you know. But thank you for paying
that price."

I wept when I read those words. This work has had a high
toll, but nothing—not one thing—could persuade me to let
my heart turn to stone. I had tasted and seen the goodness of
the Lord, and I was not willing to let anything take that hope
from me. Not trauma. Not betrayal. Not the internet. Not
abandonment. Not my own defense mechanisms. Not hardship. Not sharing my work publicly. Not getting hurt. Nothing.

It's been worth it.

Recognizing the value of keeping my heart soft has become
a profound support to me as I continue to do my own work
in compassionate resourcing. In a way, I think that's what
my friend was saying to me: Thank you for connecting to
resources, feeling the pain, setting the boundaries, tending
the wounds, and doing the work you've needed to so you
don't get hard. Because how can we be strong like water when
our innermost self is hard? It simply won't work. It requires
fierce compassion to hold the line when everything around
us wants to remake us into that which we are not.

I suspect this is what the author of Proverbs meant when

he said, "Above all else, guard your heart, for everything you do flows from it" (4:23).

Or as the Passion Translation says, "Above all, guard the affections of your heart, for they affect all that you are. Pay attention to the welfare of your innermost being, for from there flows the wellspring of life."

Of course, this is quite easy to say. Most of us love the idea of an open heart, of softness. But in reality, it's hard to hold on to that in a world that often permits—and sometimes even celebrates—brutality, violence, and harm. Often, we want to "guard the affections of [our] heart" but we don't always know how. Sometimes we will miss the mark. We will have to reimagine more than once. There is compassion and grace available to us as we flex and bend, ebb and flow in our humanity. This will be our continual work: to participate with God in creating a new way; of co-creating a life that reflects the beauty of "on earth as it is in heaven."

My dear reader, as we come to the close of our strong-like-water work, it is my deep hope that you will have every resource you need to tend to your heart and fiercely advocate to keep it soft. I also hope and pray you have felt seen and honored in these pages. Wherever you are on the flow of strength, whatever parts of your story are still in need of tending, in whatever ways you are moving toward integration and wholeness, I hope you come to know in your innermost self how valuable and loved you are. I realize this is not easy work, and I want you to know I am proud of you.

Let's keep going—honoring, hoping, believing, and healing together.

With you, dear ones.

BECOMING STRONG LIKE WATER
PRACTICING HEALING

In this last strong-like-water practice, we are going to utilize our ability to both imagine and reimagine as a way to leverage and experience strength.[8] This exercise is similar to the one in chapter 7; however, we are adapting it to create templates from what *could be.* This can be particularly helpful for those who have a history of unresolved trauma because we may not have the neurobiological framework to support the new actions we want to take. Even though we know what we're doing isn't working, we're just too overwhelmed to try taking a different path. This is where a future video may be helpful: It can bridge the gap between our current skills and what we want to happen—whether setting a limit, keeping a commitment, practicing self-care, or doing some other hard thing.

Generally, there are two main theories as to why picturing what we want to happen works. The first is that when we visualize an experience, our brain interprets it as actually occurring. Second, as we visualize the situation, our bodies react with tiny movements that cause our brain to lay down neural networks we can access when we actually move ahead with our goal.[9] The power that comes with being able to engage possibility through our imagination is incredible.

To begin, you will visualize a situation that you want to navigate successfully. Keep in mind that it's best not to use the most difficult obstacle you're facing, especially when you're beginning to learn this skill.

Now that you have this situation in mind, ask yourself, *What might success look like to me?* Try to focus on what you can control rather than on what you hope others will do or what might simply work out. For example, if you're trying to visualize successfully setting a limit with a demanding coworker, it's helpful to be as realistic about the situation as you can. Let's say you want to tell your coworker that you will no longer agree to her last-minute requests to do her work for her, which require you to stay late at the office. You know she won't take that well, so it will be important not to base success on how well she receives the limit you are setting. Instead, success should be based on your ability to implement a boundary that aligns with your integrity regardless of her response.

After deciding what success will look like, you come to the fun part: utilizing your imagination to help integrate the resources you've found supportive into the future video. Let's say that in the past, you have succumbed to your coworker's requests to pick up the slack because you wanted to avoid conflict. The question becomes: What support do you need to be able to speak up now? Perhaps you visualize yourself taking a deep breath before talking with your coworker. Perhaps you connect with an affirmation like "My voice matters."

Use the following prompts to help guide you through this practice.

1. My situation:

2. What would success look like for me in this experience?

3. What resources will I need to navigate this situation in a way that aligns with my goals and values?

RESTING IN GOD'S GOODNESS

If it feels like a helpful resource, consider the kind gaze of God toward you. Take a moment to sit with that visualization and internalize it as it feels supportive. As you do, you may wish to place a hand on your heart as you breathe, simply noticing how loved you are. Feel free to note what comes up for you as you rest in this space.

Additionally, if it feels like a beneficial resource, consider meditating on these verses:

> The Lord longs to be gracious to you; therefore he will rise up to show you compassion.
>
> ISAIAH 30:18

> I, the Lord your God, hold your right hand; it is I who say to you, "Fear not, I am the one who helps you."
>
> ISAIAH 41:13, ESV

> "With everlasting love I will have compassion on you," says the Lord, your Redeemer.
>
> ISAIAH 54:8, ESV

INTEGRATING YOUR
STRONG-LIKE-WATER WORK

As we come to the final practices for strong like water, I invite you to take a moment and, from a resourced place, journal your responses to the questions below.

1. What is your biggest takeaway from this work?

2. Where do you notice either transitional strength or integrated strength in your own life? As you consider this, what do you notice in your body? Take a moment to write what you're observing.

3. If your transitional and integrated strength were persons, what might they say to you? Do they have any words of wisdom or encouragement as you continue in your work?

4. If it feels like a support, consider the ways you have experienced your faith or the with-ness of God as a resource in this work.

5. Do you feel stuck in situational strength in any areas of your life? If so, why do you sense that might be?

6. What resources from this book resonate the most with you?

7. Who in your life can encourage you as you continue in this work?

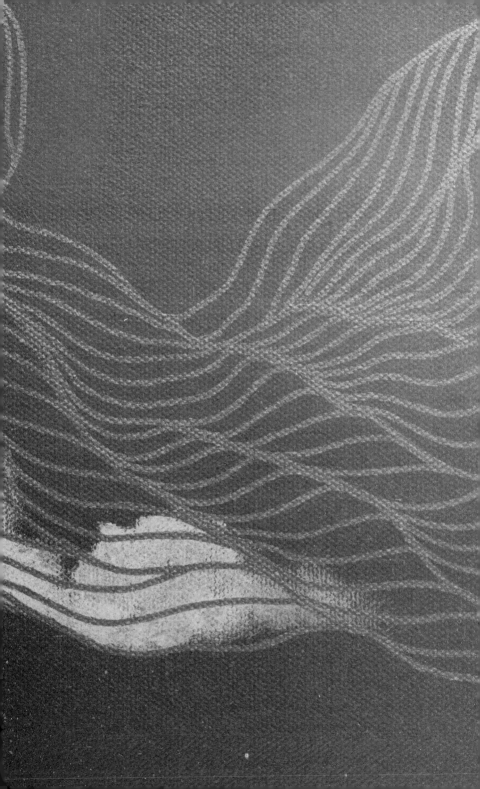

BENEDICTION

MY DEAR READER, thank you for engaging and joining me in the fierce and tender work of becoming strong like water. I pray this book has met you, supported you in places of hurt, and felt like a balm toward the parts of you that are aching for care. As you continue, may you internalize in your very flesh and bones the kind gaze of the incarnational God who fashioned you, loves you, and calls you beloved.

May you find safety in places you never dreamed and compassion in the unlikeliest of connections. May every moment of goodness you experience begin to create a reservoir of hope in your body from which you can draw whenever you need. May each of your senses be attuned to glimmers of beauty and healing wherever they are available. And when pain and difficulty come, may you have the courage and tenacity to honor them while also accessing the compassionate resources that are available to you now. In those times when you worry about being both too much and not enough, I hope you'll remember that just as your softness is a gift, so is your fire.

Reader, may you know in the depths of yourself that

healing is always, always sacred work. Nothing you do to turn with compassion toward yourself or another will go to waste because healing *is* worth the risk and the work.

And finally, my deepest prayer is that you will experience the with-ness and nearness of God—in whom all things are held together.

With you in hope,

Aundi Kolber

JANUARY 2022

ACKNOWLEDGMENTS

As many others have noted, writing a book truly cannot be done alone. And this book in particular has required much support from dear ones near and far. With that said, I owe a huge and extensive thank-you to my favorite person, my husband, Brendan. My love, words can't completely express how grateful I am to have you by my side as we've journeyed through some of the hardest hard we could have imagined. Thank you for all the ways you've showed up for me and our children. I am so much better because you exist. I love you.

To my children, Tia and Jude: Thank you for your patience and love as I've finished this manuscript. I know it's been quite the adventure, and I hope someday you'll read this book and it will remind you how magnificently God created you and how ferociously you are valued. T and J, I love you more than life itself. It is an honor to be your mama.

To my own mama: Thank you for reminding me that we can grow and heal, even when hope seems lost. Thank you for modeling bravery and helping me to know that my very blood and bones have been imbued with courage. I am grateful to be your daughter, and I love you.

To my sister, Stephanie: Thank you for teaching me my first crossover and sparking my love for basketball. You are such a treasure in my life. Thanks for your friendship, for showing up to your life, and for the many ways you've reminded me of my fierceness and belovedness—I love you to the moon and back.

To my brother Jon, thanks for all the giggles through the years and taking me to shoot hoops. To my brother Michael, I am always so grateful for your gentle heart. To my brother Anthony, thanks for the many ways you've brought me lightness, humor, and friendship. J, M, and A—I love all three of you so much.

To my in-laws Jen, Kaylin, and Jerry: Thank you for all the ways you've made our family better and more whole. I love you.

To my in-laws Barb and Chris Kolber: From helping us move across the country to providing childcare to cooking us great meals to simply encouraging us and loving us, thank you! I love you and am so grateful for you.

To my sisters-in-law, Katie, Anna, and Bethany, and your spouses: What a gift you are to me. To all my nieces and nephews: I am so excited to see you continue to grow into your God-given selves. I love you so.

To Whitney and Ryan H.; Ashley A.; Steve and Sarah C.; Alison C.; Ryan K.; Sarah; Lauren; and Chuck D.: Each of you has played such an incredibly important role in my life. I'm beyond grateful for you and your friendship. To my book club ladies— what a gift you've been to me during some heavy times. I love you! And to Hannah H.: Thanks for the many ways you've helped me stay organized!

To our wonderful friends Norm and Jenny, Dave and Amy, Scott and Brandi, and Julie and Adam: Thank you for the many ways you've loved us and held us up through the years.

To my colleagues Arielle Schwartz and Barb Maiberger, thank you for your incredibly important work. To Barb T., thanks for the many ways you've held space for me. To Robert V., Holly O., Jonathan P.,

Michael C., Dana B., Kayla C., and Laura K.—each of you has been such a support both professionally and personally. Thank you.

To my agent, Don Gates, thank you for believing in my work and for the many ways you've helped advocate on my behalf. I'm deeply grateful.

To my publishing team at Tyndale, particularly my dear friend Jillian Schlossberg for championing, stewarding, and believing in my work—I just couldn't be more grateful for you. Thanks to Kim Miller for your calm wisdom and gentle hand in shaping this manuscript; you've been such a help. To Jan Long Harris, Sarah Atkinson, Amanda Woods, Cassidy Gage, Andrea Martin, Eva Winters, Annette Hayward, and the entire Tyndale team, thank you.

To my clients and readers: Though I know I am biased, you are some of the most beautiful people I have met. Thank you for believing in the work I do and allowing me to speak to you.

And finally, to the Jesus who has held me when I couldn't hold on any longer, to the God who is profoundly with me and us: Thank You for calling me Beloved and empowering me to truly live.

NOTES

INTRODUCTION: STRENGTH IN THE WAVES

1. You can search for therapists in your area at psychologytoday.com.

CHAPTER 1: THE COST OF BEING (A CERTAIN KIND OF) STRONG

1. It is common for survivors of childhood trauma to have repressed memories of disturbing experiences. Sometimes these memories resurface; other times they do not. Either way, treatments such as somatic therapy and/or eye movement desensitization and reprocessing (EMDR) can be helpful since access to all memories isn't required for healing. For more on this, see Bessel van der Kolk, *The Body Keeps the Score* (New York: Penguin, 2014).

2. Gabor Maté (@gabormatemd), "Authenticity is a survival need," Instagram, July 11, 2021, https://www.instagram.com/p/CRMi18zs0RB/.

3. For more on how co-regulation and attunement are connected, see Deb Dana, *The Polyvagal Theory in Therapy: Engaging the Rhythm of Regulation* (New York: W. W. Norton, 2018), 124. Attunement is also understood to be a building block for healthy development and relationships. For more on this, see Daniel J. Siegel, *Mindsight: The New Science of Personal Transformation* (New York: Bantam, 2010), 27.

4. Siegel, *Mindsight*, 27.

5. When caregivers are responsive and consistent, it often creates an internal sense that conflict will move toward resolution. This is typically a sign of secure attachment. For more on this, see Diane Poole Heller, *The Power of Attachment* (Boulder, CO: Sounds True, 2019), 9.

6. I am referring again to this quote from Gabor Maté (@gabormatemd), "Authenticity is a survival need," Instagram, July 11, 2021, https://www.instagram.com/p/CRMi18zs0RB/.

7. My descriptions of fight, flight, and collapse are adapted from Arielle Schwartz and Barb Maiberger, *EMDR Therapy and Somatic Psychology*

Interventions to Enhance Embodiment in Trauma Treatment (New York: Norton, 2018), 31–32. I have also added some physical descriptions based on my experience with clients over the years.

8. The freeze response I describe here is sometimes also referred to as the "fright" stage as noted by Maggie Schauer and Thomas Elbert, "Dissociation Following Traumatic Stress: Etiology and Treatment," *Zeitschrift für Psychologie/Journal of Psychology* 218, no. 2 (2010): 109–127, https://doi .org/10.1027/0044-3409/a000018. See also Arielle Schwartz, *A Practical Guide to Complex PTSD: Compassionate Strategies to Begin Healing from Childhood Trauma* (Emeryville, CA: Rockridge Press, 2020), 74.

9. The term *fawn response* was originally coined by therapist Pete Walker. More research is needed regarding the nervous system and the fawn response; however, master psychologist Dr. Arielle Schwartz notes that the fawn response seems to span the whole range of our nervous system at various times to help us best neutralize potential threats. Consultation with Dr. Arielle Schwartz, May 20, 2021.

10. Our brains develop "from the bottom up" to prioritize breathing, heart rate, and safety. See my book *Try Softer* (Carol Stream, IL: Tyndale Refresh, 2019), 31. Practically, this means that we can have a cognitive idea that something we are experiencing is "good" or "helpful," but if our bodies are simultaneously detecting threat (whether real or perceived)—our brains will not use precious energy toward processing the goodness, but will instead ignore it in favor of helping us brace for the threat. For those who have a history of unresolved trauma, this means that their brains and bodies are constantly detecting threat in the present and thus constantly having to ignore supportive stimuli. For more on how trauma and abuse shapes brains, see Katharine Gammon, "How Neglect and Abuse Change Children's Brains—and Their Futures," Center for Health Journalism, July 19, 2017, https://centerforhealthjournalism.org/2017/07/19/how -neglect-and-abuse-change-childrens-brains-and-their-futures.

11. Experiences such as racism, poverty, and discrimination have not always been recognized as having the capacity to be traumatic; however, they absolutely can be (and whether or not they are traumatic, they are still unjust). For more on the physiology of trauma around racism, you might want to consider reading Resmaa Menakem, *My Grandmother's Hands: Racialized Trauma and the Pathway to Mending Our Hearts and Bodies* (Las Vegas: Central Recovery Press, 2017).

12. These "parts" of ourselves may be available when our trauma gets activated, but that is different than experiencing integration with that part after the trauma.

13. I first heard this quote on Brené Brown's podcast. See Brené Brown, "Strong Backs, Soft Fronts, and Wild Hearts," *Unlocking Us with Brené Brown* podcast, November 4, 2020, https://brenebrown.com/podcast/brene-on -strong-backs-soft-fronts-and-wild-hearts/.

14. Hypervigilance is connected to the activation of our sympathetic nervous system. For more, see "What Is Hypervigilance a Symptom Of?," PsychCentral, https://psychcentral.com/health/hypervigilance#signs.

15. Excessive attention to detail is connected to the activation of our sympathetic nervous system.

16. Depending on a person's trauma history, they may have a combination of hyperindependence and hyperdependence in different relationships and scenarios.

17. For more on toxic positivity, see therapist Whitney Goodman's book *Toxic Positivity: Keeping It Real in a World Obsessed with Being Happy* (New York: TarcherPerigree, 2022).

18. This phrase was originally coined by psychotherapist John Wellwood in the 1980s. He defined it as "a tendency to use spiritual ideas and practices to sidestep or avoid facing unresolved emotional issues, psychological wounds and unfinished developmental tasks." I have adapted spiritual bypassing here to reflect how I have observed it in the clients and communities I have worked with.

19. This expression likely combines fight energy, which is based in the sympathetic nervous system, with a form of dissociation in order to persevere (a stimula-tion of dorsal vagal).

20. While sarcasm can often be rooted in situational strength, it's important to distinguish that from playfulness or humor in general. Often play can be an important resource in healing.

21. Siegel, *Mindsight*, 64.

22. See the presentation by Dr. Allan Schore on YouTube, "Dr. Allan Schore on Resilience and the Balance of Rupture and Repair," PsychAlive, May 13, 2014, https://www.youtube.com/watch?v=cbfuBex-3jE&feature=youtu.be&t=1.

23. I was first introduced to this concept by Barb Maiberger at an EMDR training session in 2014. Barb also describes a version of this practice in her book *Remote Together: A Therapist's Guide to Cultivating a Sustainable Practice* (Boulder, CO: Bodymind Press, 2021), 304.

24. Arielle Schwartz, "Grounding," Center for Resilience Informed Therapy, December 12, 2017, https://drarielleschwartz.com/grounding-dr-arielle -schwartz/#.YjzCqBPMLt0.

25. This is a common resource used in trauma work. I was first introduced to this concept by Barb Maiberger at an EMDR training in 2014.

CHAPTER 2: THE NERVOUS SYSTEM: THE SACRED ROAD MAP OF OUR BODIES

1. This information is detailed in my book *Try Softer* on pages 25–27.
2. The window of tolerance interfaces with our social engagement system. I use the terms interchangeably in this chapter; however, there is some nuance to each term. *Social engagement system* speaks of the way our bodies are able to interact with other systems—using what is known as the vagal brake—in order to change or affect our state, whereas *window of tolerance* describes our abiliy to tolerate an emotional and/or physiological state while remaining regulated.
3. It was first coined by Dr. Dan Siegel; however, the work of Dr. Stephen Porges, Pat Ogden, and Dr. Arielle Schwartz has greatly influenced how I teach about it.
4. The terms *blended* and *mixed state* are both used when describing this within polyvagal theory; however, to be concise I will be using the term *blended* throughout. For a clinical description of a blended state, see Marlysa B. Sullivan et al., "Yoga Therapy and Polyvagal Theory: The Convergence of Traditional Wisdom and Contemporary Neuroscience for Self-Regulation and Resilience," *Frontiers in Human Neuroscience* (February 27, 2018): 67, https://doi.org/10.3389/fnhum.2018.00067.
5. I first learned this metaphor from Barb Maiberger when I was trained for EMDR. It is often referred to as "dual awareness" in the trauma world.
6. Polyvagal theory asserts that our nervous systems instantaneously and unconsciously detect threat, and as they do so, we move up and down a hierarchical autonomic "ladder" of potential nervous system states. Our bodies do this to help us best accommodate what we may be facing. With this in mind, our bodies tend to attempt to utilize a "pro-social" response to threat first, then they will attempt to utilize fight/flight, and if that doesn't work, they may resort to other responses such as fawning and dissociation. It's notable to remember, however, that the nervous systems of some trauma survivors have learned that a fight/flight response has never been helpful, and therefore their bodies may shift almost imperceptibly to fawning and/or dissociation.
7. *Merriam-Webster Dictionary* defines harm as "physical or mental damage." It's important to note that moving outside of our WOT can be due to someone or something causing us pain in the present, but at times it originates from past unresolved trauma that has become highly activated in the present. At other times, harm stems from both past and present factors. Depending on our unique history and experiences, the repair for various types of harm will be different.
8. A healthy or helpful amount of stress (or discomfort) is called "eustress," and when that amount goes outside of being helpful it's called "distress." These

terms were coined by endocrinologist Hans Selye in 1974 to help clarify different types of stress. For a fuller explanation, see Juliette Tocino-Smith, "What Is Eustress? A Look at the Psychology and Benefits," January 15, 2019, https://positivepsychology.com/what-is-eustress/.

9. This happens due to the way trauma is primarily stored in the right hemisphere of our amygdala, and when activated it cannot tell the difference between past and present. For more see Daniel J. Siegel, *Mindsight: The New Science of Personal Transformation* (New York: Bantam, 2010).

10. It is quite common for the threat detection system (neuroception) within survivors of childhood maltreatment to misinterpret the facial expressions, relational cues, and/or other possible indicators of threat. While researchers have not gained clarity on the exact neurobiological mechanism that influences why survivors of childhood maltreatment and/or abuse may misinterpret them, research points to the fact that normal development of accurately interpreting relational cues is interrupted. See Aislinn Sandre et al., "Childhood Maltreatment Is Associated with Increased Neural Response to Ambiguous Threatening Facial Expressions in Adulthood: Evidence from the Late Positive Potential," *Cognitive, Affective, and Behavioral Neuroscience* 18 (2018): 143–54, https://link.springer.com/article/10.3758/s13415-017-0559-z.

11. I first learned about this concept from somatic psychology, primarily the writings of Dr. Arielle Schwartz and Dr. Stephen Porges. On a physiological level, our heart rate variability (time between heart beats) is part of what nervous system flexibility means in a practical way. Our HRV is a way we measure our vagal tone, and our vagal tone speaks to the strength of our vagal brake, which we will discuss more in chapter 3.

12. Aundi Kolber (@aundikolber), Instagram, April 8, 2020.

13. This is inspired by Thomas Keating's Welcoming Prayer. See "Welcoming Prayer," Contemplative Outreach, accessed June 22, 2022, https://www.contemplativeoutreach.org/welcoming-prayer-method/.

14. For more on this, see Andrea L. Bell, "Resilience and Overwhelm: How Full Is Your 'Container'?," GoodTherapy blog, February 8, 2017, https://www.goodtherapy.org/blog/resilience-overwhelm-how-full-is-your-container-0208174.

CHAPTER 3: SAFETY IS THE MAGIC INGREDIENT

1. Unlike the other four senses, whose signals are routed first to the thalamus, scents go directly to the amygdala. This fact came from psychologist Jennifer Sweeton on a trauma training from PESI on August 10, 2021.

2. This type of response is sometimes called a body memory, which is a type of flashback that is experienced in the body in the form of emotions and sensation rather than images.

3. Deb Dana, *The Polyvagal Theory in Therapy: Engaging the Rhythm of Regulation* (New York: W. W. Norton, 2018), 35.
4. Dana, *Polyvagal Theory in Therapy*, chapter 2.
5. In his documentary *The Wisdom of Trauma*, Dr. Gabor Maté says that "safety is not the absence of threat, but the presence of connection." This pairs with polyvagal theory, which posits that for safety to be felt we need to experience cues of safety provided by co-regulation and self-regulation. This helps explain why loneliness can be dysregulating to our nervous system, even when there seems to be an absence of threat. All of these ideas taken together help us understand the larger picture of "felt safety."
6. According to polyvagal theory, as we access our ventral vagal (which is what we connect to when we are in our window of tolerance), our social engagement system comes online. For simplicity, I am using the language of WOT in tandem with the social engagement system.
7. Dana, *Polyvagal Theory in Therapy*, 28.
8. Or in polyvagal theory, what would be known as ventral vagal.
9. This comment is based on the following quote from Stephen Porges: "When working efficiently, neuroception enables a match between risk and autonomic state." See Stephen W. Porges, "The Polyvagal Theory: New Insights into Adaptive Reactions of the Autonomic Nervous System," *Cleveland Clinic Journal of Medicine* 76, supplement 2 (April 2009): S86–S90, https://doi.org/10.3949/ccjm.76.s2.17.
10. Bessel van der Kolk, *The Body Keeps the Score: Brain, Mind, and Body in the Healing of Trauma* (New York: Penguin, 2014), 352.
11. Dana, *Polyvagal Theory in Therapy*, 37.
12. Resmaa Menakem, *My Grandmother's Hands: Racialized Tauma and the Pathway to Mending Our Hearts and Bodies* (Las Vegas: Central Recovery Press, 2017), chapter 6.
13. Dana, *Polyvagal Theory in Therapy*, 28.
14. Dana, *Polyvagal Theory in Therapy*, 28.
15. Dana, *Polyvagal Theory in Therapy*, 28.
16. The vagal brake is an expression of our ventral vagal complex. There is now a way to measure the health of our vagal brake by determining our vagal tone through something called heart rate variability (HRV). The more often we learn to return to safety, the stronger our vagal tone will be, and all the strong-like-water work is designed to support this work. For more on this, see Elizabeth A. Stanley, *Widen the Window: Training Your Brain and Body to Thrive during Stress and Recover from Trauma* (New York: Avery, 2019), 86.
17. Even someone who has a well-exercised vagal brake (also known as vagal tone) can experience trauma. However, our ability to learn to co-regulate

and self-regulate can often increase our capacity and resilience as we move through difficulty.

18. For more on this, see Porges, "The Polyvagal Theory: New Insights." See also my book *Try Softer* (Carol Stream, IL: Tyndale Refresh, 2019), 77.

19. These words are inspired by Deb Dana's quote: "Trauma compromises our ability to engage with others by replacing patterns of connection with patterns of protection." See Dana, *Polyvagal Theory in Therapy*, xviii.

20. For a helpful overview of many of these principles, see Curt Thompson, *Anatomy of the Soul* (Carol Stream: Tyndale Refresh, 2010), 30–48.

21. Hara Estroff Marano, "Our Brain's Negative Bias," *Psychology Today*, June 20, 2003, https://www.psychologytoday.com/us/articles/200306/our-brains-negative-bias.

22. Dana, *Polyvagal Theory in Therapy*, xviii.

23. Arielle Schwartz, *The Complex PTSD Workbook: A Mind-Body Approach to Regaining Emotional Control and Becoming Whole* (Berkeley, CA: Althea Press, 2016), 85.

24. Chuck DeGroat, "Where Are You?," *Reformed Journal* blog, October 18, 2016, https://blog.reformedjournal.com/2016/10/18/where-are-you/.

25. DeGroat, "Where Are You?"

26. Cole Arthur Riley, *This Here Flesh: Spirituality, Liberation, and the Stories That Make Us* (New York: Convergent Books, 2022), 13.

27. This exercise was inspired by and adapted from @sensitivetherapist on Instagram, July 27, 2021.

CHAPTER 4: STRENGTH WITH CONNECTION

1. Dr. Dan Siegel calls each of us "natural born contingency detectors." This means each of us has an innate sense of when someone authentically "gets us" vs. when they are simply telling us what we want to hear. This is what I experienced with Brendan. I was introduced to this phrasing via Diane Heller in her book *The Power of Attachment: How to Create Deep and Lasting Intimate Relationships* (Boulder, CO: Sounds True, 2019). She notes that it originated in Siegel's keynote address with Diane Ackerman, "Imagining Tomorrow: Healing and Hope in the Human Age," March 28, 2015, Psychotherapy Networker Conference, Washington, DC.

2. This means that our prefrontal cortex may be partially or fully engaged and/or we may be fully or partially inside our window of tolerance.

3. For more on the neurobiology of how this happens, see chapter 4 in my book *Try Softer: A Fresh Approach to Move Us out of Anxiety, Stress, and Survival Mode—and into a Life of Connection and Joy* (Carol Stream, IL: Tyndale Refresh, 2020).

4. Deb Dana, *The Polyvagal Theory in Therapy: Engaging the Rhythm of Regulation* (New York: W. W. Norton, 2018), 40.

5. Allan N. Schore, "The Effects of Secure Attachment Relationship on Right Brain Development, Affect Regulation, and Infant Mental Health," *Infant Mental Health Journal* 22 (2001): 7–66; Allan N. Schore, "The Effects of Early Relationship Trauma on Right Brain Development, Affect Regulation, and Infant Mental Health," *Infant Mental Health Journal* 22 (2001): 201–69.

6. For more on attachment, see my book *Try Softer*, chapter 3.

7. John Bowlby pioneered the work of attachment theory and first identified three main styles: secure, avoidant, and anxious. The practical research of Mary Ainsworth further advanced this theory. See John Bowlby, *A Secure Base: Parent-Child Attachment and Healthy Human Development* (New York: Basic Books, 1988), as well as Saul McLeod, "Mary Ainsworth," *Simply Psychology*, updated 2018, https://www.simplypsychology.org/mary-ainsworth.html.

8. Disorganized attachment was not one of the original categories of attachment identified by John Bowlby but was later identified by Mary Ainsworth. Disorganized attachment is the least understood and researched of all the attachment styles. A helpful resource to learn more about this attachment style is Diane Heller, *The Power of Attachment*.

9. Amir Levine and Rachel Heller, *Attached: The New Science of Adult Attachment and How It Can Help You Find—and Keep—Love* (New York: TarcherPerigee, 2010), 125–37.

10. This is referred to as "earned secure attachment," a term originally coined by Dr. Dan Siegel.

11. James Strong, *Strong's Concordance*, s.v. "nahal," https://biblehub.com/hebrew/5095.htm.

12. James Strong, *Strong's Concordance*, s.v. "menuchah," https://biblehub.com/hebrew/4496.htm.

13. James Strong, *Strong's Concordance*, s.v. "ra'ah," https://biblehub.com/hebrew/7462.htm.

14. *The Wisdom of Trauma* documentary featuring Gabor Maté, directed by Maurizio and Zaya Benazzo, 2021.

15. This question is inspired from Barb Maiberger's advanced EMDR training on grief in 2017, where we learned to help clients create a team of allies.

CHAPTER 5: STRENGTH WITH INNER TRUST

1. This phrase is from Dr. Daniel J. Siegel's book *Mindsight: The New Science of Personal Transformation* (New York: Bantam, 2010), 19.

2. Dr. Kristin Neff's impactful book *Self-Compassion: The Proven Power of Being Kind to Yourself* (New York: William Morrow, 2011) lists "common humanity" as one of the three main ways we can access self-compassion. Though transitional strength is not the same as self-compassion, I conceptualize self-compassion as a resource that becomes possible once we move into transitional strength because we are no longer operating only from our lower brain.
3. My dear friend and fellow therapist Whitney once said this to me about fifteen years ago and I'll never forget it.
4. This statistic is from Amir Levine and Rachel Heller, *Attached: The New Science of Adult Attachment and How It Can Help You Find—and Keep—Love* (New York: TarcherPerigee, 2010), 8–9. The authors estimate that roughly 50 percent of the population are secure, 20 percent are anxious, 25 percent are avoidant, and 5 percent are disorganized.
5. Oftentimes, unprocessed pain and/or trauma will cause us to feel strongly identified with ourselves at various ages. This happens because unprocessed pain is located in the right hemisphere of our amygdala (which cannot tell the difference between the past and the future), and when the pain is activated, we can lose a sense of our current age. Ideally, however, we aim to connect with that sense of pain (or younger self) while also remaining connected with our present-day self.
6. Diane Poole Heller, *The Power of Attachment* (Boulder, CO: Sounds True, 2019), 70.
7. In their book *Attached* (page 127), Levine and Heller speak to the ways that people with an avoidant attachment style utilize deactivating strategies to repress connection even when they actually do want to connect.
8. Heller, *Power of Attachment*, 83.
9. For more on implicit memories, see Siegel, *Mindsight*, 149, as well as my book *Try Softer*, 98–99.
10. Heller, *Power of Attachment*, 83.
11. Heller, *Power of Attachment*, 114–15.
12. This phrase is coined by Diane Heller in *The Power of Attachment*.
13. It is common for people to have more than one "younger self" as they engage inner child work. However, to be concise, I'm only referring to one "younger self" here.
14. This is a widely regarded idea in psychology that is influenced and inspired by the work of Dr. Dan Siegel, Dr. Arielle Schwartz, Barb Maiberger, Dr. Allan Schore, and Dr. Gabor Maté.
15. Self-compassion is a concept highly popularized by the research of Dr. Kristin Neff. In her book *Self-Compassion*, she notes that three distinct pillars—(1) mindfulness; (2) common humanity; and

(3) self-kindness—make self-compassion possible. You can also read more about this in chapter 9 of *Try Softer*.

CHAPTER 6: STRENGTH WITH GOODNESS

1. To my surprise, about six months after I wrote this story, Brendan and I moved within a few hours of the cottage.
2. Deb Dana, *The Polyvagal Theory in Therapy: Engaging the Rhythm of Regulation* (New York: Norton, 2018), 68.
3. Though it may seem counterintuitive, initially goodness may feel triggering for some trauma survivors. This is typically because in the past, resources of goodness were paired with something harmful. This is one reason the pacing of the nervous system matters because it allows a person to adjust as they learn to experience goodness without the fear or dread connected to it.
4. Dr. Alison Cook shared her thoughts on this topic in an Instagram post on June 2, 2021.
5. Ryan Kuja shared his thoughts in a Facebook post on April 17, 2021. His full quote is, "Resurrection is in our cells and in the wiring of our autonomic pathways. Resurrection is in the brain's neuroplasticity and the capacity of the broken bone and the broken heart to mend. Resurrection is baked into the makeup of the human body and the universe itself."
6. "Practice resurrection" is the last line of the poem "Manifesto: The Mad Farmer Liberation Front," which is found in Wendell Berry, *The Country of Marriage* (Berkeley, CA: Counterpoint, 2013), 14, https://cals.arizona.edu/~steidl/Liberation.html.
7. The word *disturbance* is often used as a broad term to cover various categories of trauma and/or other experiences that may affect our nervous system in the work of EMDR or other trauma therapies.
8. Dr. Arielle Schwartz notes that trauma is typically stored in our brain's right hemisphere (and the right hemisphere is more likely to hold negative perceptions), whereas the left hemisphere of our brain is more likely to hold positive emotions. When trauma is activated, a person is unable to access the adaptive resources from their left hemisphere, which is why the trauma remains stuck. EMDR facilitates the integration of these two hemispheres so that the trauma can experience repair and closure. For more on the ways that EMDR can facilitate healing, see Arielle Schwartz, "How Does EMDR Therapy Work?," Center for Resilience Informed Therapy, October 10, 2017, https://drarielleschwartz.com/how-does-emdr-therapy-work-dr-arielle-schwartz/#.Ym2PgPPMIq0.
9. The term *dual attention stimulation* (DAS) is used in conjunction with the term *BLS*. For brevity, I will use BLS for our discussion going forward.

10. See Definition of Terms, s.v. "Bilateral Stimulation Therapies (BLSTs)," Parnell Institute, accessed April 30, 2022, https://parnellemdr.com /definition-of-terms/.

11. Laurel Parnell, *Tapping In: A Step-by-Step Guide to Activating Your Healing Resources through Bilateral Stimulation* (Boulder, CO: Sounds True, 2008), 17.

12. The theory behind bilateral stimulation is that it seems to mimic what our brain does in REM sleep, which is when our unconscious taps into deep processing. Additionally, there is evidence that it "decreases the vividness, somatic arousal, and emotional intensity associated with traumatic memories," according to Arielle Schwartz and Barb Maiberger, *EMDR Therapy and Somatic Psychology* (New York: W. W. Norton, 2018), 52.

13. Parnell, *Tapping In.*

14. These resources have been inspired by and adapted from the work of EMDR trainer and therapist Barb Maiberger, as well as the work of Dr. Laurel Parnell in her book *Tapping In.*

15. I originally learned about the importance of a somatic vocabulary at a training which integrates EMDR with Somatic psychology in July 2017. This list is one I've compiled as I've worked with clients.

CHAPTER 7: STRENGTH WITH EMOTIONAL FLEXIBILITY

1. Psychologist and executive coach Susan David says this type of flexibility "allows you to be in the moment, changing or maintaining your behaviors to live in ways that align with your intentions and values. The process isn't about ignoring difficult emotions and thoughts. It's about holding those emotions and thoughts loosely, facing them courageously and compassionately." See Susan David, *Emotional Agility: Get Unstuck, Embrace Change, and Thrive in Work and Life* (New York: Avery, 2016), 11.

2. Daniel J. Siegel, *Mindsight: The New Science of Personal Transformation* (New York: Bantam, 2010), 17.

3. For more on this, see my book *Try Softer* (Carol Stream, IL: Tyndale Refresh, 2019), pages 180–84.

4. "Emodiversity: A Mix of Emotions Is Healthiest?," *Discover* magazine, October 13, 2014, https://www.discovermagazine.com/mind/emodiversity -a-mix-of-emotions-is-healthiest, emphasis mine. An abstract of the study is found at Jori Quoidbach et al., "Emodiversity and the Emotional Ecosystem," *Journal of Experimental Psychology General* 143, no. 6 (December 2014): 2057–66, https://pubmed.ncbi.nlm.nih.gov/25285428/.

5. I first learned this concept at an advanced training for EMDR by Barb Maiberger in 2015 and 2017.

6. Though early therapy sessions typically include discussing a client's history, there are methods available that allow us to minimize how deeply someone goes into their history so that it is not re-traumatizing.

7. Peter Levine, *Waking the Tiger: Healing Trauma* (Berkeley, CA: North Atlantic Books, 1997), 238.

8. I first learned this concept at an advanced training for EMDR by Barb Maiberger in 2015 and 2017. For more on this concept see also my book *Try Softer*, 126–28.

9. On a neurobiological level, this resource activates her brain's left hemisphere (which tends toward "positive" states) with the right hemisphere (which tends toward negative perceptions). Additionally, the sense of calm helps Erica engage her vagal brake. In a way, it's as if the fear is talking to the resource, which expands Erica's capacity to deal with the challenge.

10. Both terms are often used when polyvagal theory is discussed. To be concise, I will be using *blended state* throughout. For a more thorough discussion regarding the neurobiology of blended states, see https://www.ncbi.nlm .nih.gov/pmc/articles/PMC5835127/. You may also consider reading more here: Stephen W. Porges, "Vagal Pathways: Portals to Compassion," in *The Oxford Handbook of Compassion Science*, ed. Emma M. Seppälä (New York, NY: Oxford University Press, 2017), 189–202.

11. Arielle Schwartz, "Mind-Body Therapies for Vagus Nerve Disorders," Center for Resilience Informed Therapy, May 23, 2018, https://drarielleschwartz .com/vagus-nerve-disorders-dr-arielle-schwartz/#.YUIb255Kg6E.

12. For more information on the ways these experiences can be harmful, see this overview of the Adverse Childhood Experiences study from the National Conference of State Legislatures at https://www.ncsl.org/research/health /adverse-childhood-experiences-aces.aspx.

13. I first learned this language from Barb Maiberger at a training for EMDR and have found it to be invaluable.

14. For more, see Francine Shapiro, *Eye Movement Desensitization and Reprocessing (EMDR) Therapy: Basic Principles, Protocols, and Procedures*, 3rd ed. (New York: Guilford, 2018).

15. The practices that follow were adapted from Dr. Arielle Schwartz, "Mind-Body Therapies for Vagus Nerve Disorders," blog at Center for Resilience Informed Therapy, May 23, 2018, https://drarielleschwartz.com/vagus -nerve-disorders-dr-arielle-schwartz/#.Yv6vF3bMKUk. Dr. Schwartz notes that these practices are beneficial because they help strengthen our vagal tone. For other ideas on strengthening vagal tone, see my book *Try Softer*, 217.

16. For more on the Internal Family Systems (IFS) model see, see Richard C. Schwartz, *Introduction to the Internal Family Systems Model* (Oak Park, IL:

Trailheads Publications, 2001). Or for an overview of IFS that integrates a Christian faith perspective, see Alison Cook and Kimberly Miller, *Boundaries for Your Soul: How to Turn Your Overwhelming Thoughts and Feelings into Your Greatest Assets* (Nashville: Nelson, 2018).

17. Cook and Miller, *Boundaries for Your Soul*, 26. They also note these qualities are based on IFS's seven *c*'s.

18. Typically when discussing this work from a polyvagal perspective, we would say ventral vagal complex (VVC) versus window of tolerance. Though they are not completely interchangeable, they overlap significantly. With this in mind, I am using the WOT in order to keep it consistent with the other parts of *Strong like Water*.

19. For more on the ways the ventral vagal allows us to access blended states, see Marlysa B. Sullivan et al., "Yoga Therapy and Polyvagal Theory: The Convergence of Traditional Wisdom and Contemporary Neuroscience for Self-Regulation and Resilience," *Frontiers in Human Neuroscience* 12 (2018): 67, https://www.ncbi.nlm.nih.gov/pmc/articles/PMC5835127/.

20. Sullivan et al., "Yoga Therapy and Polyvagal Theory."

21. "READ: Youth Poet Laureate Amanda Gorman's Inaugural Poem," CNN, January 20, 2021, https://www.cnn.com/2021/01/20/politics/amanda-gorman-inaugural-poem-transcript/index.html.

22. Soong-Chan Rah, *Prophetic Lament: A Call for Justice in Troubled Times* (Downers Grove, IL: IVP, 2015), 21.

23. Gabor Maté, "When the World Won't Hold Us: Finding Agency in the Suffering," *Psychotherapy Networker*, September/October 2020, https://www.psychotherapynetworker.org/magazine/article/2489/when-the-world-wont-hold-us/212e4cc7-ac6a-444f-8c3f-bf1de0d0defd.

24. Henri Nouwen, *The Return of the Prodigal Son: A Story of Homecoming* (New York: Doubleday, 1994), 129.

25. Though I name emotion here, I don't advocate for utilizing this practice to process past trauma on your own. However, sometimes our emotions can be stuck because past trauma has made all experience of feelings seem unsafe. With this in mind, you may wish to use this resource to practice putting the support you would need in a future video in order to help you move through emotions that come up in your everyday life. (See pages 175–76.)

26. This is a part of EMDR protocol designed by Francine Shapiro. However, much of the way I've learned to use future videos has been adapted through Francine Shapiro's work as well as training under Barb Maiberger, MA, LPC.

27. This first appeared in my book *Try Softer* on page 214.

28. I find fascinating the science explaining why visualization (and thus a future video) may work. In her book *Remote Together: A Therapist's Guide to*

Cultivating a Sustainable Practice (Boulder, CO: Bodymind Press, 2021), 284–85, Barb Maiberger offers two reasons visualization can be helpful: "The first theory is Symbolic Learning which hypothesizes that when you see yourself doing an activity, the brain lays down a neural pathway. This pathway contains information on the movement's coordination, such as brushing your teeth, driving a car, or even doing something fancy like a double pirouette in ballet. The more you repeat this movement in your imagination, the more automatic and easier it becomes to perform. This neural pathway begins to support the muscle memory, which is essential for athletes, dancers, musicians, public speakers, teachers, and, yes, clients in therapy regulating their nervous systems. The second theory, Psychoneuromuscular Learning, states that when you visualize an activity, the brain will send signals to the muscles to contract, which fires neurons so that you can complete the action. Essentially, when you visualize the movement of doing a double pirouette, the brain is firing neurons as if you're doing this activity even though you just imagine it."

CHAPTER 8: STRENGTH WITH MOVING THROUGH

1. My first exposure to understanding that our bodies are designed to literally metabolize and move through pain came by being trained in EMDR in 2014. I am indebted to Barb Maiberger MA, LPC, for her fabulous work as a trainer in the EMDR field.
2. In trauma work, having an experience that is deeply disturbing or that otherwise overwhelms our nervous system's capacity to cope has the potential to become a type of trauma. It's important to note, however, that not all disturbing experiences become trauma—largely based on what type of support and resources are present during and after the experience.
3. My thoughts here are based on what Dr. Allan Schore calls a mother's and/or caregiver's role as "psychobiological regulators" for children who are not yet able to process experiences or emotions in a way that allow their bodies to remain integrated. Thus the role of a caregiver is to assist in providing regulation. See Allan N. Schore, *The Science of the Art of Psychotherapy* (New York: Norton, 2012). Additionally, the work of Dr. Dan Siegel, Dr. Stephen Porges, and Deb Dan deeply enrich this idea through the lenses of interpersonal neurobiology and polyvagal theory.
4. Peter Levine, *Waking the Tiger: Healing Trauma* (Berkeley, CA: North Atlantic Books, 1997), chapter 17.
5. These questions are based on the ways that adults intuitively develop this type of internal secure base when they have experienced secure attachment.

It's important to remember that even if you haven't experienced this in childhood, it's possible to experience earned secure attachment.

6. Levine, *Waking the Tiger*, 99–100.

7. As we discussed in chapter 3, our neuroception is constantly at work helping us discern how to utilize our energy and protective responses.

8. I'm referring to the presence of a secure, attuned presence to help them widen their window of tolerance.

9. Other aspects of "completing the stress cycle" are addressed in Emily Nagoski and Amelia Nagoski, *Burnout: The Secret to Unlocking the Stress Cycle* (New York: Ballantine, 2019).

10. For a more thorough explanation on completion, see Chris Walling, "Psychotherapy for Your Body: The Role of Somatic Psychology Today," GoodTherapy, June 5, 2017, https://www.goodtherapy.org/blog/psychotherapy-for-your-body-role-of-somatic-psychology-today-0605174. See also Levine, *Waking the Tiger*.

11. For an overview of this, see Peter A. Levine, *In an Unspoken Voice: How the Body Releases Trauma and Restores Goodness* (Berkeley, CA: North Atlantic Books, 2010), 22–23.

12. Though experiences such as chronic illness and/or chronic pain are much too multifaceted to connect to only one source, researchers are finding that the inflammation of a prolonged stress response from toxic stress and/or unprocessed trauma (including the emotions connected to those events) may create a stronger correlation to experiencing chronic illness/pain. Importantly, this does not place blame on someone experiencing chronic illness or pain, but it does help us understand ways to potentially work with our bodies in treating it. For an overview of this connection, see "Are Childhood Trauma and Chronic Illness Connected?" Healthline, https://www.healthline.com/health/chronic-illness/childhood-trauma-connected-chronic-illness#What-the-research-says.

13. Francine Shapiro, the creator of EMDR, theorized that our bodies have an adaptive information processing (AIP) system that, when given enough support, allows a person's body to have the intuition to know what is needed to heal trauma. For more on this, see Francine Shapiro, *Eye Movement Desensitization and Reprocessing (EMDR) Therapy: Basic Principles, Protocols, and Procedures*, 3rd ed. (New York: Guilford, 2018).

14. In many ways, the completion of the stress cycle is the opposite of trauma.

15. My thoughts here are again based on the adaptive information processing (AIP) theory proposed by Francine Shapiro.

16. For more on this, see Arielle Schwartz and Barb Maiberger, *EMDR Therapy and Somatic Psychology: Interventions to Enhance Embodiment in Trauma Treatment* (New York: W.W. Norton, 2018), 49–55.

17. Psychiatrist Curt Thompson notes that the right brain experiences sensations and then the left brain works to narrate or "prove" what is being felt. Thus, when we "move through" a stress cycle, our left brain narrates the reality that this experience feels completed in our body. For more on how the left brain and the right brain operate, see Curt Thompson, *Anatomy of the Soul: Surprising Connections between Neuroscience and Spiritual Practices That Can Transform Your Life and Relationship* (Carol Stream, IL: Tyndale Refresh, 2010), 10, 31–38.

18. Vincent J. Felitti et al., "Relationship of Childhood Abuse and Household Dysfunction to Many of the Leading Causes of Death in Adults: The Adverse Childhood Experiences (ACE) Study," *American Journal of Preventive Medicine* 14, no. 4 (May 1998): 245–58, https://doi.org/10.1016/S0749-3797(98)00017-8.

19. Robert Frost, "A Servant to Servants," in *North of Boston* (New York: Henry Holt, 1915), 66.

20. Somatic psychology, and particularly the work of Dr. Peter Levine, explores the many ways that suppressing movement after trauma can affect us.

21. Arielle Schwartz, *The Post-Traumatic Growth Guidebook: Practical Mind-Body Tools to Heal Trauma, Foster Resilience and Awaken Your Potential* (Eau Claire, WI: PESI Publishing, 2020), 23.

22. Dr. Dan Siegel notes that our ability to empathize with the experience of others is based in our ability to travel our own circuits. In order to do this, a person needs to have some connection with their insula, which then relays information from their mirror neurons down into their body, allowing them to "resonate" with others. When we are disconnected from our body and ourself, we are unable to experience this type of resonance.

23. I first learned about this concept from Dr. Arielle Schwartz, and this practice is an adaption from one she provides at Arielle Schwartz, "Healing PTSD: Mind and Body in Trauma Treatment," Center for Resilient Informed Therapy blog, August 4, 2020, https://drarielleschwartz.com/healing-ptsd-mind-and-body-in-trauma-treatment-dr-arielle-schwartz/#.YfL5AVjMITU.

24. Bessel van der Kolk, *The Body Keeps the Score: Brain, Mind, and Body in the Healing of Trauma* (New York: Penguin, 2014), 51–55.

25. Levine, *Waking the Tiger*, 27.

26. Anecdotally I have heard that Dr. Peter Levine recommends, "When in doubt, voo it out."

CHAPTER 9: STRENGTH WITH INTEGRATION

1. Dr. Kristin Neff describes self-compassion as "a caring force" that has both a tender and fierce side. For more see Kristin Neff, *Fierce Self-Compassion:*

How Women Can Harness Kindness to Speak Up, Claim Their Power, and Thrive (Harper Wave: New York, 2021).

2. I first heard this phrase from the book *Becoming Safely Embodied: A Guide to Organize Your Mind, Body and Heart to Feel Secure in the World* by Deirdre Fay.

3. James Strong, *Strong's Concordance*, s.v. "metanoia," https://biblehub.com/greek/3341.htm.

4. One example in which *metanoia* and *epistrephō* are paired is Acts 3:19: "Repent, then, and turn to God, so that your sins may be wiped out, that times of refreshing may come from the Lord."

5. James Strong, *Strong's Concordance*, s.v. "epistrephō," https://biblehub.com/greek/1994.htm.

6. Sharon Salzberg, "Meditation Is about Recovering and Starting Again," Mindful, February 7, 2019, https://www.mindful.org/meditation-is-about-recovering-and-starting-again/.

7. Practice inspired by a line from Naomi Goodlet, "Protect and Replenish Your Energy Meditation," Insight Timer, accessed June 13, 2022, https://insighttimer.com/naomigoodlet/guided-meditations/protect-and-replenish-your-energy.

CHAPTER 10: STRENGTH WITH REIMAGINING

1. For a helpful resource on the many ways neuroplasticity is connected to grace, see Curt Thompson, *Anatomy of the Soul: Surprising Connections between Neuroscience and Spiritual Practices That Can Transform Your Life and Relationship* (Carol Stream, IL: Tyndale Refresh, 2010), 139.

2. See Romans 8:22.

3. James Baldwin, "As Much Truth as One Can Bear," *New York Times*, January 14, 1962 (emphasis mine).

4. Steve Carter, *The Thing beneath the Thing: What's Hidden Inside (and What God Helps Us Do about It)* (Nashville: W Publishing, 2021).

5. "TU110: Story Follows State—Investigating Polyvagal Theory with Guest Deb Dana," *Therapist Uncensored* podcast, December 5, 2019, https://therapistuncensored.com/episodes/tu110-story-follows-state-investigating-polyvagal-theory-with-guest-deb-dana/.

6. Martin Luther King Jr. spoke these words during a 1963 speech in Detroit.

7. Osheta Moore, *Dear White Peacemakers: Dismantling Racism with Grit and Grace* (Harrisonburg, VA: Herald Press, 2021), 96.

8. This practice has been adapted from Francine Shapiro's future videos from EMDR protocol.

9. See Barb Maiberger, *Remote Together: A Therapist's Guide to Cultivating a Sustainable Practice* (Boulder, CO: Bodymind Press, 2021), 284.

ABOUT THE AUTHOR

AUNDI KOLBER is a licensed professional counselor (LPC), speaker, and author of the groundbreaking book *Try Softer* and its companion, *The Try Softer Guided Journey*. Aundi is the owner of Kolber Counseling, LLC, established in 2009. In addition to her MA in community counseling, she has received additional training in her specialization of trauma- and body-centered therapies, including the highly researched and regarded eye movement desensitization and reprocessing (EMDR) therapy.

Aundi is passionate about the integration of faith and psychology, and is a sought-after expert and speaker in both faith and secular settings. She has appeared on podcasts such as *The Lazy Genius* with Kendra Adachi, *Typology*, and *The Next Right Thing* with Emily P. Freeman. Aundi reaches an audience of over 50,000 via email and social media. You can find her at @aundikolber on Instagram and Twitter or at aundikolber.com.

As a survivor of trauma and a lifelong learner, Aundi brings hard-won knowledge around the work of change, the power of redemption, and the beauty of experiencing God *with* us in our pain. She is happily married to her best friend, Brendan, and is the proud mom of Matia and Jude.

Also available from Aundi Kolber . . .

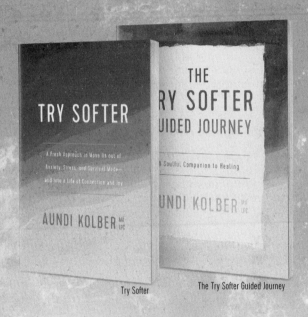

Try Softer

The Try Softer Guided Journey

Trying softer is sacred work. This is what we were made for: a living, breathing, moving, feeling, connected, beautifully incarnational life.

Available wherever books are sold.